Vaccine Research and Development to Advance Pandemic and Seasonal Influenza Preparedness and Response

Lessons from COVID-19

Enriqueta Bond, Kanta Subbarao, and Hoda Soltani, *Editors*

Committee on Vaccine Research and Development Recommendations for Advancing Pandemic and Seasonal Influenza Preparedness and Response

Board on Global Health

Health and Medicine Division

A Consensus Study Report of

The National Academies of
SCIENCES · ENGINEERING · MEDICINE
and
NATIONAL ACADEMY OF MEDICINE

THE NATIONAL ACADEMIES PRESS
Washington, DC
www.nap.edu

THE NATIONAL ACADEMIES PRESS 500 Fifth Street, NW, Washington, DC 20001

This activity was supported by a contract between the National Academy of Sciences and the Office of Global Affairs with the U.S. Department of Health and Human Services. Any opinions, findings, conclusions, or recommendations expressed in this publication do not necessarily reflect the views of any organization or agency that provided support for the project.

International Standard Book Number-13: 978-0-309-08781-0
International Standard Book Number-10: 0-309-08781-3
Digital Object Identifier: https://doi.org/10.17226/26282
Library of Congress Catalog Number: 2021950193

Additional copies of this publication are available from the National Academies Press, 500 Fifth Street, NW, Keck 360, Washington, DC 20001; (800) 624-6242 or (202) 334-3313; http://www.nap.edu.

Printed in the United States of America

Suggested citation: National Academies of Sciences, Engineering, and Medicine. 2022. *Vaccine research and development to advance pandemic and seasonal influenza preparedness and response: Lessons from COVID-19*. Washington, DC: The National Academies Press. https://doi.org/10.17226/26282.

The National Academies of

SCIENCES • ENGINEERING • MEDICINE

The **National Academy of Sciences** was established in 1863 by an Act of Congress, signed by President Lincoln, as a private, nongovernmental institution to advise the nation on issues related to science and technology. Members are elected by their peers for outstanding contributions to research. Dr. Marcia McNutt is president.

The **National Academy of Engineering** was established in 1964 under the charter of the National Academy of Sciences to bring the practices of engineering to advising the nation. Members are elected by their peers for extraordinary contributions to engineering. Dr. John L. Anderson is president.

The **National Academy of Medicine** (formerly the Institute of Medicine) was established in 1970 under the charter of the National Academy of Sciences to advise the nation on medical and health issues. Members are elected by their peers for distinguished contributions to medicine and health. Dr. Victor J. Dzau is president.

The three Academies work together as the **National Academies of Sciences, Engineering, and Medicine** to provide independent, objective analysis and advice to the nation and conduct other activities to solve complex problems and inform public policy decisions. The National Academies also encourage education and research, recognize outstanding contributions to knowledge, and increase public understanding in matters of science, engineering, and medicine.

Learn more about the National Academies of Sciences, Engineering, and Medicine at **www.nationalacademies.org.**

The National Academies of
SCIENCES • ENGINEERING • MEDICINE

COMMITTEE ON VACCINE RESEARCH AND DEVELOPMENT RECOMMENDATIONS FOR ADVANCING PANDEMIC AND SEASONAL INFLUENZA PREPAREDNESS AND RESPONSE[1]

ENRIQUETA BOND (*Co-Chair*), Founding Partner, QE Philanthropic Advisors
KANTA SUBBARAO (*Co-Chair*), Director, Collaborating Centre for Reference and Research on Influenza, World Health Organization
MARIA ELENA BOTTAZZI, Associate Dean, National School of Tropical Medicine; Professor of Pediatrics and Co-Director, Texas Children's Center for Vaccine Development, Baylor College of Medicine; Co-Chair, Vaccines and Therapeutics Taskforce, Lancet Commission on COVID-19
REBECCA J. COX, Professor of Medical Virology and Head of the Influenza Centre, University of Bergen and Haukeland University Hospital
ANNETTE FOX, Senior Research Scientist, Collaborating Centre for Reference and Research on Influenza, World Health Organization
FLORIAN KRAMMER, Professor of Microbiology, Department of Microbiology, Icahn School of Medicine at Mount Sinai
GRACE M. LEE, Professor of Pediatrics, Stanford University School of Medicine
JOHN C. MARTIN (*until March 30, 2021, deceased*), former Chief Executive Officer and Executive Chairman, Gilead Sciences
JOSHUA M. SHARFSTEIN, Professor of the Practice in Health Policy and Management, Johns Hopkins Bloomberg School of Public Health
MILAGRITOS D. TAPIA, Professor, Pediatrics, University of Maryland School of Medicine

Study Staff

HODA SOLTANI, Study Director
EMILIE RYAN-CASTILLO, Senior Program Assistant
ELIZABETH ASHBY, Research Associate
HANNAH K. COLLINS, Research Associate
PATRICIA A. CUFF, Senior Program Officer
JULIE A. PAVLIN, Senior Director, Board on Global Health

Consultant

MAARTJE WOUTERS, Science Writer

[1] See Appendix B, Disclosure of Unavoidable Conflict of Interest.

In Memoriam

John C. Martin, Ph.D., M.B.A.
1951–2021

Reviewers

This Consensus Study Report was reviewed in draft form by individuals chosen for their diverse perspectives and technical expertise. The purpose of this independent review is to provide candid and critical comments that will assist the National Academies of Sciences, Engineering, and Medicine in making each published report as sound as possible and to ensure that it meets the institutional standards for quality, objectivity, evidence, and responsiveness to the study charge. The review comments and draft manuscript remain confidential to protect the integrity of the deliberative process.

We thank the following individuals for their review of this report:

RAFI AHMED, Emory University
RUSSEL BASSER, Seqirus
NORMAN BAYLOR, Biologics Consulting
PHIL DORMITZER, Pfizer Vaccine
MICHAEL OSTERHOLM, University of Minnesota
PETER PALESE, Mount Sinai
KATHERINE POEHLING, Wake Forest School of Medicine
TED ROSS, University of Georgia

Although the reviewers listed above provided many constructive comments and suggestions, they were not asked to endorse the conclusions or recommendations of this report nor did they see the final draft before its release. The review of this report was overseen by **ANN M. ARVIN,** Stanford University School of Medicine, and **ALASTAIR J. WOOD,** Vanderbilt University. They were responsible for making certain that an independent examination of this report was carried out in accordance with the standards of the National Academies and that all review comments were carefully considered. Responsibility for the final content rests entirely with the authoring committee and the National Academies.

National Academy of Medicine

Advancing Pandemic and Seasonal Influenza Vaccine Preparedness and Response Series

This study, Vaccine Research and Development to Advance Pandemic and Seasonal Influenza Preparedness and Response: Lessons from COVID-19, provides recommendations on how to leverage the knowledge gained from the COVID-19 pandemic to optimize research and development for future pandemic and seasonal influenza vaccines. It is one of four studies conducted under the Advancing Pandemic and Seasonal Influenza Vaccine Preparedness and Response Initiative, which explores how the scientific and technological breakthroughs throughout the COVID-19 pandemic could inform and advance future pandemic and seasonal influenza vaccine preparedness and response efforts.

The three companion studies to this study examine how the lessons learned from COVID-19 around vaccine distribution and supply chain contingencies, public health interventions and countermeasures, and global coordination, partnerships, and financing could be best utilized to improve the development and distribution of future pandemic and seasonal influenza vaccines. Together, the four studies present a path toward better preparedness in addressing pandemic and seasonal influenza.

Launched by the National Academy of Medicine with support from the Office of Global Affairs, U.S. Department of Health and Human Services, the Advancing Pandemic and Seasonal Influenza Vaccine Preparedness and Response Initiative acknowledges that influenza is here to stay. The unprecedented scope of this initiative allowed for international experts to look at this issue from multiple angles and provide recommendations that set out a pathway to more effective influenza vaccines worldwide. Driven by international cooperation, this independent initiative provides a platform to highlight why we need to act as a global community to better prepare for pandemic and seasonal influenza.

Acknowledgments

The committee has been honored and privileged to be able to contribute to this important effort and wishes to acknowledge the valuable contributions and assistance of many individuals who shared their expertise. The Statement of Task was developed by an international committee of experts assembled by the National Academy of Medicine. Many thanks to many area experts who volunteered their time to present to the committee and provided invaluable insights to inform the recommendations in this report. In this vein, we extend our thanks to Ben Cowling (University of Hong Kong); Barney Graham (NIH); Rita Helfand (WHO); Robert Johnston (BARDA); David Kaslow (PATH); Jerome Kim (International Vaccine Institute); Nicole Lurie (CEPI); Peter Marks (FDA); Kathleen Neuzil (University of Maryland – Center for Vaccine Development); Julie Ostrowsky (CIDRAP); Rino Rappuoli (GlaxoSmithKlein); Nadine Rouphael (Emory Vaccine Center); and Melanie Saville (CEPI). Finally, we thank the outstanding support and work of the National Academies of Sciences, Engineering, and Medicine project staff for overseeing the assembly of our committee and the details of this report. We deeply appreciate the work of Hoda Soltani, Study Director; Emilie Ryan-Castillo, Senior Program Assistant; Elizabeth Ashby, Research Associate; Hannah Collins, Research Associate; Patricia Cuff, Senior Program Officer; and Julie Pavlin, Senior Director, Board on Global Health. This project would not be possible without the support of the Office of Global Affairs at the U.S. Department of Health and Human Services.

Preface

The National Academy of Medicine (NAM) has established an international committee in coordination with the U.S. Department of Health and Human Services' Office of Global Affairs (OGA) to inform and facilitate efforts to advance global influenza pandemic preparedness. This international committee will provide OGA with an iterative, interactive multidisciplinary process for assessing the global effect that capabilities, technologies, processes, and policies developed for COVID-19 pandemic could have on pandemic and seasonal influenza global preparedness and response, especially regarding vaccine development. As part of the NAM initiative, the National Academies of Sciences, Engineering, and Medicine are carrying out four concurrent consensus studies. As one of the four work streams of this effort, our committee examined the technological and scientific advances achieved during the global response to COVID-19 and other outbreaks to distill lessons learned for vaccine research, development, and manufacturing, including the use of platform technologies to recommend strategies to harness the science, technology, policy, and practice required to improve global influenza pandemic preparedness and response.

In the 1980s as the United States mounted a response to address the harsh realities of the HIV/AIDS pandemic, Nobel laureate Joshua Lederberg warned that the public and political leadership of the United States needed to seriously address emerging infectious diseases and their potential for devastating epidemics. In 1992 the Institute of Medicine (IOM) published the landmark report *Emerging Infections: Microbial Threats to Health in the United States*, which pointed to major challenges for the public health and medical care communities in detecting and managing infectious disease outbreaks and monitoring the prevalence of endemic diseases. A decade later *Microbial Threats to Health: Emergence, Detection, and Response*, underscored the revolution in globalization of all spheres including political, economic, cultural, technological, and informational—a new global environment where infectious agents could migrate with the internationalization of goods and people.

The severe acute respiratory syndrome (SARS), the Middle East respiratory syndrome, and Ebola serve as classic examples for how diseases can emerge and reemerge with unexpected fluctuations in different parts of the world. Fortunately, each was controlled before it grew into a pandemic. Then SARS coronavirus 2 (SARS-CoV-2) emerged, causing the COVID-19 pandemic, with dramatic loss of human life and devastating social and economic disruption worldwide. In October 2020, Cutler and Summers estimated the costs of COVID-19 in the United States at $16 trillion. As of August 2021, the Johns Hopkins University map notes that globally there have been nearly 190 million cases, more than 4 million recorded deaths, though some estimate total deaths may be as high as 16 million, and nearly 3.6 billion courses of vaccine administered. While an unprecedented number of vaccines has been developed, much more needs to be done to reach the nearly 8 billion human beings on Earth. The pandemic continues as variants have emerged.

Most experts believe that an influenza pandemic is inevitable given (1) the circulation of different influenza A subtypes in animals, (2) current global circulation of two A subtypes in humans, and (3) the ability of the viruses to mutate and reassort. In the early 20 century, the Spanish influenza caused an estimated 50 million deaths worldwide. Additional influenza pandemics in 1957, 1968, and 2009 claimed lower numbers of lives but still had an enormous impact on global human health and the economy. For this reason, for several years, governments, philanthropy, and global organizations have focused much attention to influenza pandemic preparedness planning. These efforts certainly facilitated the scientific and public health response to COVID-19, but they fell short, as we have seen with the inequities and the inability to vaccinate all. In the process of responding to COVID-19, lessons learned can be deployed to help the world respond better to the next influenza pandemic.

The main lesson has been that, given the astonishing and devastating costs to human life and the global economy, many more resources need to be sustainably invested in continued research, platform development for new influenza vaccines, and the regional capacity to research, manufacture, and distribute vaccines. Unprecedented cooperation and coordination among the different academic, government, industry, philanthropic, and global organizations have facilitated COVID-19 vaccine development and provided models for the future, but more needs to be done to ensure that low- and middle-income countries also benefit and that we do not lose momentum in preparing ourselves for a future influenza pandemic.

Enriqueta Bond, *Co-Chair*
Kanta Subbarao, *Co-Chair*
Committee on Vaccine Research and Development
Recommendations for Advancing Pandemic and Seasonal
Influenza Preparedness and Response

Contents

Boxes and Figures

BOXES

FIGURES

Acronyms and Abbreviations

Ad26	adenovirus serotype 26
BARDA	Biomedical Advanced Research Development Authority
CDC	U.S. Centers for Disease Control and Prevention
CEPI	Coalition for Epidemic Preparedness Innovations
CIDRAP	Center for Infectious Disease Research and Policy
CMC	chemistry, manufacturing, and control
COBRA	computational optimized broadly reactive antigens
CONSISE	Consortium for the Standardization of Influenza Seroepidemiology
COVID-19	coronavirus disease 2019
CVD	Centre pour le Developpement des Vaccins
DNA	deoxyribonucleic acid
EMA	European Medicines Agency
EUA	Emergency Use Authorization
FDA	U.S. Food and Drug Administration
FLUCOP	Standardization and Development of Assays for Assessment of Influenza Vaccine Correlates of Protection
GAP	Global Action Plan

GISAID	Global Initiative on Sharing All Influenza Data
GISRS	Global Influenza Surveillance and Response System
HA	hemagglutinin
HHS	U.S. Department of Health and Human Services
HI	hemagglutinin inhibition
HIC	high-income country
ICMRA	International Coalition of Medicines Regulatory Authorities
IHR	International Health Regulations
IP	intellectual property
LMIC	low- and middle-income country
mAb	monoclonal antibody
MDCK	Madin-Darby canine kidney
MERS	Middle East respiratory syndrome
NA	neuraminidase
NAM	National Academy of Medicine
NIAID	National Institute of Allergy and Infectious Diseases
NIH	National Institutes of Health
NK	natural killer
OWS	Operation Warp Speed
PRR	pattern recognition receptor
QIV	quadrivalent inactivated vaccine
R&D	research and development
SARS	severe acute respiratory syndrome
SARS-CoV-2	severe acute respiratory syndrome coronavirus 2
SPEAC	Safety Platform for Emergency vACcines
TIV	trivalent inactivated vaccine
TTS	thrombosis with thrombocytopenia syndrome
UIV	universal influenza vaccine
VAERS	Vaccine Adverse Event Reporting System

VE	vaccine effectiveness
VSD	Vaccine Safety Data Link
WHO	World Health Organization
YODA	Yale Open Data Access

Summary

The global response to the COVID-19 pandemic has led to the emergence of new capabilities, technologies, processes, and policies for responding to the threat of major infectious diseases. While today, COVID-19 dominates the conversation around vaccines, the critical threat of both seasonal and pandemic influenza remains. Accordingly, at the request of the U.S. Department of Health and Human Services, the National Academy of Medicine (NAM) within the National Academies of Sciences, Engineering, and Medicine (the National Academies) undertook a series of four studies to examine how lessons learned from the response to COVID-19 and the resulting advances can best be applied to improve preparedness for and response to seasonal and pandemic influenza. The following report represents the findings, conclusions, and recommendations of one of these studies, focusing on vaccine research and development (R&D).

As many as 650,000 respiratory-related deaths per year worldwide result from influenza. Although vaccination is the most successful and cost-effective strategy for the prevention and control of seasonal influenza, uptake of vaccines is generally low, owing in part to a lack of availability and competing health priorities in many low- and middle-income countries (LMICs). Both global and domestic efforts, including the U.S. National Influenza Vaccine Modernization Strategy 2020–2030 and the World Health Organization (WHO) Global Influenza Strategy 2019–2030, articulated a need for more effective influenza vaccines, as well as modern manufacturing technologies that are adaptable and can be scaled to meet demand during a pandemic. The rapid development of COVID-19 vaccines has demonstrated what can be achieved when there is extensive data sharing and researchers have the necessary resources and novel technologies to conduct and apply their research. This report documents the key drivers of success in this model and how it might be applied to optimize vaccine R&D to support the prevention and control of both seasonal and pandemic influenza. Given the scale of this threat, the committee urges expedient development of 4.15–8.31 billion courses of influenza vaccine to be distributed globally in a timely and equitable manner.

ABOUT THIS STUDY

The NAM initiative is focused on how to improve (1) the global design, composition, clinical trials, production, scale-up, and regulatory approval for influenza vaccines; (2) distribution of the vaccines; and (3) postapproval surveillance for adverse events. The initiative was spearheaded by a committee of domestic and international experts representing a range of sectors (e.g., government, academia, industry, civil society, international public health organizations) and a variety of salient disciplines. The international committee's role included developing the Statements of Task for the four concurrent National Academies studies, each to be conducted by an ad hoc committee of experts in the respective topic. The present report details the findings of an ad hoc committee charged with identifying a framework, informed by the response to COVID-19, for optimizing vaccine research, development, and delivery in response to pandemic and seasonal influenza. The committee's findings address four dimensions of vaccine R&D: (1) basic and translational science, (2) clinical science, (3) manufacturing science, and (4) regulatory science. These findings served as the basis for the committee's recommendations within each of these four dimensions, directed at both U.S. and international actors, for developing a rapid capability to produce and distribute enough vaccine doses for the global population in a timely and equitable manner worldwide in response to both pandemic and seasonal influenza.

BASIC AND TRANSLATIONAL SCIENCE

Continuous funding streams are vital for vaccine R&D. While funding is typically available during pandemics, it is significantly lacking during interpandemic periods. This lack of funding often stalls R&D progress made during pandemic periods and leaves the world ill prepared for the next one. The vast majority of influenza vaccines are inactivated virus vaccines grown in eggs, with limited use of cell culture platforms. Production of pandemic vaccines would rely on the egg-based platform. Despite having the advantage of being an established process, there are limitations, in particular concerning the production time. As seasonal egg-based influenza vaccines have low to moderate efficacy and require annual updates due to antigenic drift, significant funding is necessary to develop novel platforms and technologies that may lead to more efficacious vaccines. A priority focus for future basic and clinical research on influenza vaccines should be the investigation into how to overcome issues associated with viral antigenic drift for seasonal vaccines. COVID-19 has resulted in a paradigm shift in vaccine technology, presenting benefits of other vaccine platforms for fast development of pandemic vaccines and the improvement of seasonal vaccine effectiveness. When considering novel platforms for further development, other factors such as expanding manufacturing capacity, feasibility of scale-up in LMIC, effectiveness, speed, and cost must also be addressed. For each new platform, standardized assays, reagents, and animal models will be needed in addition to research on surrogate markers of protection for those vaccines not inducing hemagglutination-inhibiting antibodies. Furthermore, there is a need for research into novel adjuvants, and for licensing and capacity building for the manufacturing of adjuvants. These research efforts would facilitate making rational choices regarding platforms for vaccine development that take into account the effectiveness, the speed of development and production, and the costs. Investments in pandemic preparedness are not only critical for public health, they are economically beneficial. The cost of responding to a pandemic is estimated be $570 billion annually, while investments in pandemic preparedness would cost just $4.5 billion annually. Funding pandemic preparedness will allow a framework for international collaboration to be built, providing vital support for global vaccine development.

Recommendations

Recommendation 2-1: The U.S. Department of Health and Human Services, through the National Institute of Allergy and Infectious Diseases, the Biomedical Advanced Research and Development Authority, and the U.S. Department of Defense, as well as other corresponding governmental and funding agencies domestically and abroad, should invest, proportionate to the enormous costs of pandemics, in basic and translational research to reveal a diverse array of influenza vaccines, using different platforms, viral targets, adjuvants, and delivery systems. This will allow selection of the candidates most fit for purpose to be brought to authorization and sufficient production and distribution to optimize the control of influenza across diverse settings and phases of pandemics and epidemics.

Recommendation 2-2: The World Health Organization should advocate and coordinate with multilateral stakeholders (e.g., the Coalition for Epidemic Preparedness Innovations), governments, funding agencies, the vaccine industry, and philanthropic organizations to build global capacity for robust and internationally comparable preclinical, clinical, and immunological assessments of influenza vaccine candidates, including novel candidates that use innovative structures, targets, and delivery systems to potentially broaden or improve protection.

Recommendation 2-3: International research networks (e.g., the National Institutes of Health/U.S. Centers for Disease Control and Prevention funding networks) supported by governments and funding agencies, the World Health Organization, and the vaccine industry should support, carefully plan, and conduct multi-center international clinical trials and field studies to compare emerging vaccines with standard vaccines in, among others, geographically, demographically, and immunologically diverse populations to inform rational and situation-based use and manufacture of an extended array of vaccines.

Recommendation 2-4: National regulators should engage with the vaccine industry and academic researchers in the development, standardization, and implementation of innovative assays to evaluate vaccines that induce immunity through mechanisms other than strain-specific neutralizing hemagglutination-inhibiting antibodies in order to reach consensus on the validation of these assays that will allow approval or licensure of influenza vaccines based on a broader range of assays that reflect induction of immunity.

CLINICAL SCIENCE

Research for the next generation of influenza vaccines requires extensive investment in clinical development. However, given the costly nature of conducting clinical studies, many industries see little incentive. The expansion of clinical trials globally, particularly in LMICs, will decrease the risk of such large investments and fill the clinical funding gap. Despite the significant impact of influenza in LMICs, many lack seasonal vaccine programs owing to both a lack of funding and a lack of perceived urgency. To highlight the urgency of such seasonal influenza programs to local governments, burden-of-disease studies and cost–benefit analyses are needed. Furthermore, population-based studies of vaccine effectiveness for novel vaccines need to capture the diversity of racial, ethnic, socioeconomic, age, and medical conditions within and across countries. To control for other variables that may bias effectiveness, electronic medical records can be used to provide context on comorbidities.

Clinical studies of influenza vaccines need to represent the diversity of the population studied, and high-risk groups should be prioritized in early studies so that vaccines can be made available to the most at-risk populations first. Clinical research into vaccines using novel platforms will require postapproval vaccine effectiveness studies and safety surveillance on a global scale; data sharing is essential for this purpose, as are survey-based approaches to monitor postapproval vaccine safety. Increasing involvement of LMICs in both clinical trials and distribution capacities is essential and will require a coordinated global pharmacovigilance system. For this purpose, lessons can be learned from community-engaged work that collaborates and partners with the local community.

Recommendations

Recommendation 3-1: The World Health Organization, in collaboration with national public health agencies (e.g., the U.S. Centers for Disease Control and Prevention, the European Centre for Disease Prevention and Control, the China Center for Disease Control and Prevention, and the Africa Centres for Disease Control and Prevention) should conduct burden-of-disease studies in low- and middle-income countries to understand factors such as the health and economic burden of influenza illness and barriers to immunization in adult, pregnant, and pediatric populations to ensure development of infrastructure and capacity needed for pandemic vaccine development and implementation. Cost–benefit analyses should include additional economic productivity losses caused by delayed access to a vaccine in a pandemic.

Recommendation 3-2: The International Coalition of Medicines Regulatory Authorities and the World Health Organization, in partnership with national regulatory (e.g., the U.S. Food and Drug Administration and the European Medicines Agency) and public health agencies (e.g., the U.S. Centers for Disease Control and Prevention, the European Centre for Disease Prevention and Control, the China Center for Disease Control and Prevention, and the Africa Centres for Disease Control and Prevention) should invest, on a global level, in data infrastructure and capacity building to conduct real-time sentinel site surveillance of vaccine safety and effectiveness of different vaccine products deployed for use in epidemics and pandemics in diverse populations (e.g., age group, gender, race/ethnicity, geographic, presence of comorbidities, preg-

nancy, and socioeconomics), including a plan to ensure coordination, collaboration, and data sharing across these sentinel surveillance sites.

Recommendation 3-3: The International Coalition of Medicines Regulatory Authorities and the World Health Organization (Global Advisory Committee on Vaccine Safety) should ensure international coordination and collaboration on the timely and transparent review of vaccine safety data during epidemics and pandemics to support real-time decision making about the use of vaccines. Safety data should be made available to support country-level benefit–risk assessments, particularly for low- and middle-income countries relying on regional data from sentinel sites conducting safety surveillance.

MANUFACTURING SCIENCE

As the majority of the world's vaccine manufacturing capacity is located in high-income countries (HICs), they have the advantage of early access to pandemic vaccines. Early access to vaccines combined with the funds required to purchase them leads to the type of vaccine nationalism seen during the COVID-19 pandemic. Prioritizing the expansion of manufacturing capacity in LMICs will help avoid the delayed rollout of vaccines in LMICs that occurs when only HICs are afforded access. This would not only benefit LMICs, but could also benefit the entire world as it expedites the time to control the pandemic and limits the spread of virus variants. The global network of influenza centers of excellence could guide the effort to combat vaccine nationalism, in which countries make deals with manufacturers and ensure the supply to their own population first, resulting in global vaccine inequity, by increasing collaboration and expanding to ensure capacity building in LMICs. Additional factors causing delays in vaccine manufacturing during a pandemic include shortages of supplies such as lab reagents, consumables, and raw materials caused by increased demand and reduced production and delivery of raw materials. A current bottleneck for the production of pandemic influenza vaccines is the steady supply of embryonated chicken eggs. Exploration of novel platforms for vaccine production can complement conventional vaccine production and lower the risk of supply chain shortages. However, proprietary issues have not been resolved for novel platforms, which may be a limiting factor in expanding global manufacturing capacity. Public-sector investments and improvements to data-sharing infrastructure will increase vaccine manufacturers' ability to mobilize quickly during the next pandemic. Financial aid provided by public investment may also incentivize vaccine manufacturers to assume more risk in building infrastructure to accommodate vaccine R&D in preparation for the next impending influenza pandemic.

Recommendations

Recommendation 4-1: The U.S. Department of Health and Human Services and the World Health Organization should develop a plan for a sufficient and self-sustainable global supply of influenza vaccines for pandemics. This includes

- **Convening, supporting, and encouraging multi-national, public, and private vaccine manufacturers to benchmark, prioritize, and harmonize influenza vaccine manufacturing; and**
- **Enhancing and expanding support of the global influenza vaccine manufacturing network, creating manufacturing hubs for greater collaboration, and building capacity to address challenges in manufacturing in low- and middle-income countries.**

Recommendation 4-2: Vaccine manufacturers should take a risk-based approach to pandemic influenza preparedness. This approach would be most effective if incentivized, and could include

- **Participating during research and development, data sharing, technology adoption, and training activities with international partners;**
- **Expanding internal capacity to assess the production needs and their risks;**
- **Using scientific evidence to design strategies to reduce risks (e.g., World Health Organization prequalification, licensing, and marketing); and**
- **Formalizing technology transfer (scale-up and scale-out) activities, taking into consideration timelines and the outcomes for equitable costs, access, and distribution.**

REGULATORY SCIENCE

The COVID-19 pandemic is a model for the future of regulatory science. Regulatory systems developed clear requirements and collaborated with industry partners to share data. This helped to conduct overlapping preclinical and early clinical phase studies, rapidly increasing the speed with which the COVID-19 vaccines were developed. Nevertheless, the process can be improved to accelerate the development of pandemic influenza vaccines. More data sharing between vaccine manufacturers during the preclinical and clinical development of vaccines for pandemics would be beneficial. Regulators must develop guidelines for how to conduct preclinical and early clinical trials during interpandemic periods and develop pathways for rapid review of vaccines for pandemic strains. Additionally, clear regulations for the development of seasonal vaccines are needed, including correlates of protection, efficacy, and safety. If vaccine manufacturers use international standards for testing efficacy, it will ensure all vaccines meet set standards for correlates of protection while also streamlining development.

The COVID-19 pandemic also highlighted the importance of transparent communications with the public. The lack of transparency and clear communication from both vaccine manufacturers and government agencies contributed to vaccine hesitancy in many populations. Preventing vaccines from becoming politicized and properly communicating the risks and benefits, as well as safety information, could have instilled trust in the vaccines. To combat these issues, regulators should commit to releasing clinical trial data for independent analysis. Additionally, national regulators could collaborate with scientific leaders to establish coordinated communications with the public to help convey differences in vaccine recommendations across different countries and regions.

Recommendations

Recommendation 5-1: The U.S. Food and Drug Administration and other national regulators (e.g., European Medicines Agency) working with the scientific community and pharmaceutical industry should enhance comprehensive guidance for the development of influenza vaccines on novel platforms through Emergency Use Authorization to full licensure. This guidance should provide pathways for seasonal and pandemic influenza.

Recommendation 5-2: The U.S. Food and Drug Administration and other national regulators (e.g., European Medicines Agency) should commit to transparency in the oversight of clinical trials, review of data, authorization, and approval of pandemic influenza vaccines, including the release of facility inspection findings, clinical trial protocols, and clinical data that are the basis of decision making. Regulators should convene independent advisory committees to systematically review data, make recommendations, and build public understanding and confidence prior to the authorization or approval of novel vaccines.

Recommendation 5-3: The World Health Organization and the International Coalition of Medicines Regulatory Authorities should encourage and support the coordination between regulatory and public health agencies (e.g., the U.S. Centers for Disease Control and Prevention, the European Centre for Disease Prevention and Control, the China Center for Disease Control and Prevention, and the Africa Centres for Disease Control and Prevention) when announcing different decisions

on the same or similar vaccines, to explain the different underlying circumstances and judgments.

Recommendation 5-4: Vaccine manufacturers should adopt a code of conduct for press releases and other communications regarding vaccine trial results and other matters that emphasizes the critical role of regulatory review.

1

Introduction

Throughout 2020 and 2021, the global response to COVID-19 demonstrated the importance of vigilance and preparedness for infectious diseases. In this context, there was a marked demand placed on vaccine research and development (R&D), with researchers, federal agencies, public health institutions, manufacturers, and regulators being rapidly mobilized to develop an effective vaccine as quickly as possible. Throughout this process, many opportunities and hurdles were identified that can inform the development of a conceptual framework for limiting the spread of future viral outbreaks, including pandemic influenza. The U.S. National Influenza Vaccine Modernization Strategy 2020–2030 (HHS, 2020) and the World Health Organization (WHO) Global Influenza Strategy 2019–2030 (WHO, 2019), have both called for improving influenza vaccines with respect to both effectiveness and scalable manufacturing technologies. As demonstrated throughout the response to COVID-19, the process of R&D of novel vaccines can be significantly optimized when stakeholders are provided with the resources and technologies needed to support research and when data are shared in real time (Kinsella et al., 2020). This report will identify the most important drivers of success in this model and provide recommendations for using those findings to support vaccine R&D for prevention and control of both pandemic and seasonal influenza outbreaks.

This report is the product of one of four studies conducted under an initiative carried out by the National Academy of Medicine (NAM) within the National Academies of Sciences, Engineering, and Medicine at the request of the U.S. Department of Health and Human Services' Office of Global Affairs. The purpose of this initiative was to use lessons learned from the response to the COVID-19 pandemic to advance vaccine preparedness for pandemic and seasonal influenza. The NAM convened an international committee of domestic and global experts who met to discuss the key issues that arose during the COVID-19 response and to identify considerations for the development of a framework for preparedness for the next pandemic, both domestically and globally. The discussions of this international committee served as the basis for the statements of task for the ad hoc committees charged with conducting the four concurrent National Academies consensus studies.

The present report was produced by the Committee on Vaccine Research and Development Recommendations for Advancing Pandemic and Seasonal Influenza Preparedness and Response, convened to identify opportunities for optimizing vaccine R&D processes in the event of an influenza pandemic, and to determine whether those opportunities could be used to inform the development of seasonal and universal influenza vaccines. The full charge to the committee responsible for this report is provided in Box 1-1. The committee included 10 members with academic and professional expertise in immunology, virology, vaccine manufacturing, and vaccine surveillance, as well as other related focus areas. The committee biographies are provided in Appendix A. Regrettably, one committee member passed away during the study.

BOX 1-1
Statement of Task

An ad hoc committee under the auspices of the National Academies of Sciences, Engineering, and Medicine will examine the technological and scientific advances achieved during the global response to COVID-19 and other outbreaks in vaccine research, development, and manufacturing, including the use of platform technologies, and recommend strategies to harness the science, technology, policy, and practice required to improve global influenza pandemic preparedness and response.

Specifically, the committee will:

1. Assess how lessons from COVID-19 and other prior epidemics have changed the research and development (R&D) ecosystem, and explore how these advances could be applied to pandemic and seasonal influenza planning, including innovative trial design approaches, regulatory approval mechanisms, and R&D capacity in resource-limited settings.
2. Distinguish pandemic-level response from seasonal influenza vaccine development and delivery, identify overlapping regulatory and policy concerns, and review the need for novel vaccine development platforms beyond traditional processes (i.e., egg-based vaccines).

BOX 1-1 Continued

3. Discuss the implications of the existing seasonal influenza response ecosystem on future influenza pandemics and consider how emerging technologies can be applied to manage seasonal or pandemic influenza outbreaks.
4. Recommend actions to strengthen and diversify the use of vaccine production facilities and novel vaccine technologies, including platform technologies (e.g., cell-based, recombinant, nucleic acid, viral vectors, and other synthetic technologies), and business strategies that could be sustainably and rapidly adapted to address multiple threats.
5. Consider the effects of issues such as viral drift, repeat immunization effects, seasonal influenza vaccine effectiveness, and intellectual property upon the technical, regulatory, and policy feasibility of recommended actions.
6. Recommend ways to build capacity for accelerated vaccine development and delivery against pandemic influenza viruses, and discuss the applicability of rapid-response procedures for seasonal influenza outbreaks.
7. Consider mechanisms to better coordinate and integrate R&D processes for newly developed vaccines with cohesive vaccine distribution and postapproval surveillance efforts. These considerations include streamlining vaccine and drug discovery, clinical testing, intellectual property management, and other international policy barriers that may impede or delay development.

STUDY APPROACH AND SCOPE

This study is intended to address the need to optimize influenza vaccine technology based on current capabilities, a need identified in the 2019–2030 WHO Global Influenza Strategy (WHO, 2019), the 2020–2030 U.S. National Influenza Vaccine Modernization Strategy (HHS, 2020), and other documents. This report presents the findings of the committee, based on discussions during a series of 10 meetings that occurred over a span of 4 months, March through August 2021. During its first meeting, the committee decided that its charge would best be met by focusing on the following four dimensions of vaccine R&D with a vision of supporting the rapid development of between 4.15 and 8.31 billion doses of influenza vaccine globally in a timely and equitable manner: (1) basic and translational science, (2) clinical science, (3) manufacturing science, and (4) regulatory science. The committee would like to emphasize the importance of building adequate capacity in these four dimensions to ensure global preparedness for the next impending influenza outbreak.

The first seven committee meetings included open sessions during which speakers presented information relevant to the committee's charge. Meeting themes were developed based on one of the above four dimensions. All public meeting agendas can be found in Appendix D. The open sessions were followed by closed sessions during which the committee reflected on key findings, conclusions, and recommendations relating to the speakers' presentations, as well as the meeting topic at hand. The 8th, 9th, and 10th meetings focused on arriving at committee consensus on outlines developed following the prior meetings, which were used by the committee and study staff to write this report.

This report is intended to provide an overview of a myriad of complex issues defined in the committee's Statement of Task (see Box 1-1); it makes no claim to providing comprehensive or systematic examination of all the available evidence on these issues. Figure 1-1 shows how each major element of the Statement of Task maps to the chapters of the report.

The content of this report was informed by the extensive expertise of the committee members, which was applied in formulating recommendations for improving influenza vaccine R&D. The findings, recommendations, and conclusions in this report also reflect evidence and accounts related to the COVID-19 pandemic that were published prior to August 2021, such as peer-reviewed journal articles, case studies, and news media articles. It should be noted that this study was initiated and carried out while the COVID-19 response was actively under way; thus, the literature available on vaccine R&D at that time may not reflect the full breadth of the growing evidence base. To circumvent such limitations, the committee relied heavily on expert accounts provided by the many speakers at its open sessions who provided key insights about vaccine R&D efforts led by various organizations in response to COVID-19, which helped to ensure that the committee had a good understanding of developments in R&D capacity as they occurred.

BACKGROUND

Previous pandemics were caused by influenza A viruses. The influenza pandemic in 1918–1919, caused by an H1N1 virus with genes of avian origin, is the largest pandemic recorded and is estimated to have caused 50 million deaths (Johnson and Mueller, 2002; Taubenberger and Morens, 2006). In 1957, the world experienced an H2N2 pandemic that was estimated to have caused 1.1 million excess deaths (Viboud et al., 2016). In 1968 a pandemic was caused by an H3N2 virus strain. This virus contained two genes from an avian virus and six genes from the 1957 H2N2 virus (Kawaoka et al., 1989). This pandemic resulted in an estimated 1 million deaths (CDC, 2019b).

The 2009 influenza pandemic was caused by a novel influenza A H1N1 virus that originated in pigs. The first cases were identified in February 2009 in Mexico (Hsieh et al., 2011). Two months later, the first U.S. cases were identified when two pediatric cases in southern California were reported to the U.S. Centers for Disease Control and Prevention (CDC, 2009). On April 25, WHO declared a public health emergency of

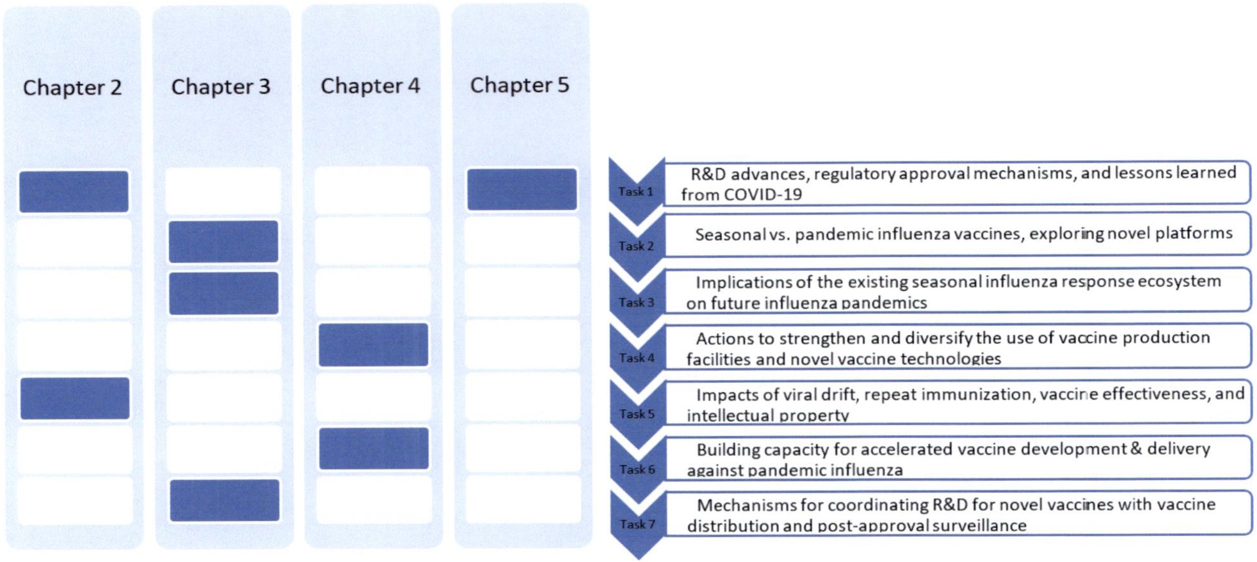

FIGURE 1-1 Mapping the major elements of the committee's Statement of Task to the chapters of this report.
NOTES: The committee will address seven major themes, outlined above in their corresponding chapters. Chapter 2 will address tasks 1 and 5; Chapter 3 will address tasks 2, 3, and 7; Chapter 4 will address tasks 4 and 6; and Chapter 5 will also address task 1.

international concern and activated the International Health Regulations (IHR) that were developed after the severe acute respiratory syndrome coronavirus (SARS) outbreak in 2003. On June 11, 2009, WHO declared a pandemic. The first vaccine virus candidates were developed a month after the public health emergency was declared, and vaccine seed strains were made available within weeks (CDC, 2019c). However, it took months for the vaccine to be manufactured and distributed, and by then, the peak was over, and the effects of the vaccine were limited. While the response was much more rapid in terms of vaccine development than what was seen during COVID-19, this pandemic showed that despite an early decision to develop vaccines, their manufacturing and distribution were too slow to limit the spread of the first wave of the virus (WHO, 2011). As of August 10, 2021, the recorded COVID-19 death toll was 4.3 million (LePan, 2021) but is estimated to be as high as 16 million. Figure 1-2 shows a history of global pandemics throughout history.

This section provides brief background information on the following:

- influenza virus and its effects on humans,
- viral antigenic drift and shift and the implications for influenza vaccine development,
- the landscape of influenza vaccine platforms,
- the effectiveness of seasonal influenza vaccines,
- the potential for developing a universal vaccine, and
- vaccine development in the context of the COVID-19 pandemic.

Chapter 2 delves into several of these topics in greater detail.

The Influenza Virus and Its Effects on Humans

The influenza virus is a segmented, negative-sense RNA virus that can be divided into four types: A, B, C, and D. Influenza types A and B cause seasonal epidemics and influenza A viruses cause sporadic pandemics. Influenza A viruses are further classified into subtypes, based on the antigenicity of the surface glycoproteins hemagglutinin (HA) and neuraminidase (NA). To date, 18 HA and 11 NA subtypes have been discovered (CDC, 2019a), of which viruses containing 3 HA (H1, H2, and H3) and 2 NA (N1 and N2) subtypes have caused epidemics in humans (Taubenberger and Morens, 2010). The virion's envelope also contains proteins that serve as ion channels (M2). The matrix protein (M1) provides structure to the virion, and within the virion, the segmented viral RNA is localized, bound to nucleoprotein and polymerase proteins (Gómez-Puertas et al., 2000).

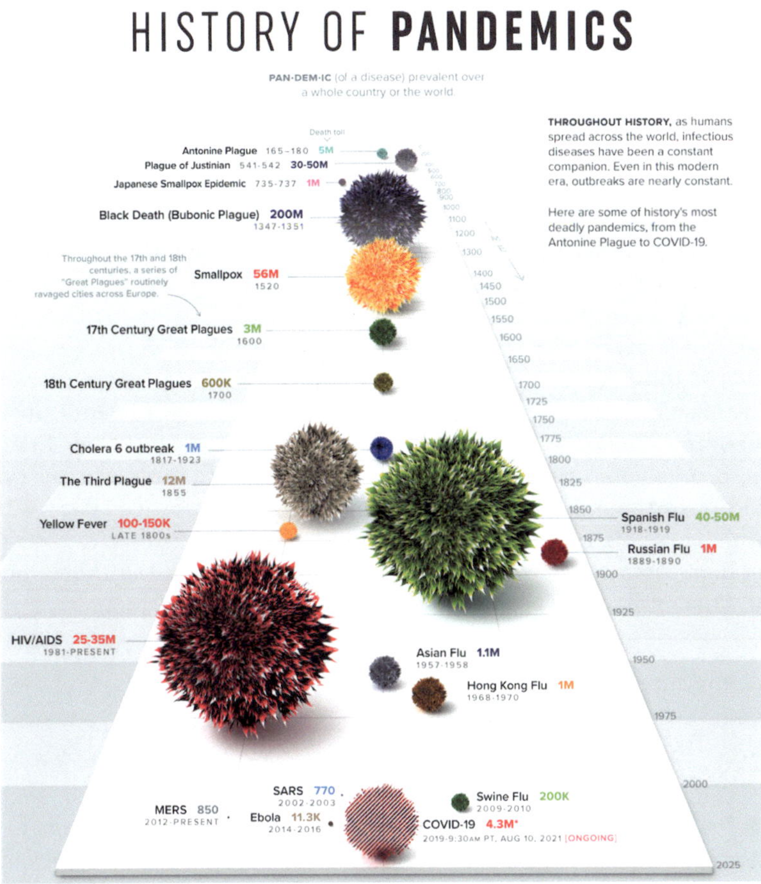

FIGURE 1-2 A history of global pandemics.
SOURCE: LePan, 2021.

Disease Caused by Influenza Viruses

The influenza virus HA attaches to the terminal α-sialic acid on the surface of the host cell and this strong binding initiates the endocytosis process (Luo, 2012). A reduction in the pH in the endosome allows the viral membrane to fuse with the host membrane; these processes are mediated by the M2 ion channel and HA. The fusion results in the release of the eight RNA viral segments into the nucleus. The RNA segments are translocated to the nucleus where they are transcribed and replicated (Luo, 2012). mRNA is transported back into the cytoplasm for translation and virion RNA segments exit the nucleus and are transported to the cell surface where new progeny virions assemble and bud.

After infection with an influenza virus, respiratory disease generally occurs within 1 to 4 days, and is characterized by a sudden onset of fever, (dry) cough, headache, muscle and joint pain, severe malaise, sore throat, and other respiratory symptoms. Symptoms peak on day 2 or 3 after infection and resolve in most cases within 9 days. Viral shedding peaks at day 2 and lasts an average of 4.8 days (Carrat et al., 2008).

In general, influenza is a self-limited illness (Ghebrehewet et al., 2016; Paules and Subbarao, 2017). Symptoms can, in severe cases, lead to pneumonia and death. Severe disease occurs worldwide in an estimated 3–5 million cases every year, resulting in 290,000–650,000 deaths (Iuliano et al., 2018; Jha et al., 2020; WHO, 2021c). Most of the severe cases and deaths occur in groups at high risk of complications of influenza, including children under the age of 5, during pregnancy, people older than 65 years, people with chronic diseases, and patients with immunosuppressive conditions or taking immunosuppressive drugs (Ortiz et al., 2018; WHO, 2021b). These high case numbers result in associated health care costs also being high at an estimated $2.0–$5.8 billion annually in the United States alone (Yan et al., 2017).

Immune Response to Natural Influenza Infection

Given that the incubation period of influenza is short, acute effects as induced by the innate immune response are essential to curb infection. Viral RNA can be recognized by pattern-recognition receptors (PRRs), such as toll-like receptors (Zhu et al., 2021). The activation of PRRs results in the production of proinflammatory cytokines and type I interferons, resulting in the inhibition of viral replication in host cells. Alveolar macrophages play an important role in the innate immune response and limit the spread of the virus by phagocytosis of infected cells. Dendritic cells present antigen to $CD4^+$ and $CD8^+$ T cells to stimulate adaptive cellular responses and can exert cytolysis (interferon killer dendritic cells).

The adaptive immune response forms the second line of defense against viral infection, consisting of humoral and cellular responses. The humoral response includes the production of IgA, IgM, and IgG antibodies that are mainly directed against HA and NA. A proportion of the antibodies directed against HA can neutralize virus infectivity by inhibiting the attachment to the receptor and viral entry, while the antibodies against NA inhibit its enzymatic activity resulting in reduced viral spread. Additionally, natural killer (NK) cells can recognize and lyse infected cells bound to antibodies, a process called antibody-dependent cell cytotoxicity. Antibodies directed against M2 protein are produced to a limited extent, and antibodies directed against nucleoproteins may result in complement-mediated cytotoxicity (Sedova et al., 2019).

Cellular immune responses consist of both $CD4^+$ and $CD8^+$ T cells (Jameson et al., 1999). $CD4^+$ T cells mainly function as helper cells, producing cytokines that stimulate B cell responses (humoral, Th2 response) and promote cellular responses (Th1 response). The main activity of $CD8^+$ T cells is as cytolytic T lymphocytes, which are activated in lymphoid tissues by antigen-presenting cells, recruiting these cells to the infection site. Cytolytic T lymphocytes kill virus-infected cells by producing and releasing perforins and granzymes, or by inducing apoptosis through the Fas/FasL pathway. Additionally, these cells also produce a series of cytokines that promote antigen presentation by stimulation of major histocompatibility complex molecule expression (Janway et al., 2001).

Viral Antigenic Drift and Shift and Implications for Vaccine Development

Influenza viruses are characterized by their ability to rapidly undergo antigenic changes caused by mutations in the antibody-binding sites of the HA and NA viral surface proteins, a process called antigenic drift. The virus acquires mutations because the viral RNA-dependent RNA polymerase does not have proofreading activity, resulting in a high error rate causing mutations in the genes and proteins (Drake, 1993). The HA is also under positive selection from immune pressure, resulting in mutations in key antigenic sites that allow the virus to escape neutralization by antibodies induced by prior infection or vaccination. Additionally, antigenic shift may occur when two viruses coinfect a cell. Coinfection results in reassortment of gene segments, giving rise to new gene constellations and introduction of novel gene segments, resulting in a novel virus that has the potential to cause a pandemic (Lopez and Legge, 2020).

Because of the pandemic and seasonal risks, it is essential that circulating influenza viruses are closely monitored. The WHO Global Influenza Surveillance and Response System (GISRS) is a worldwide surveillance network that monitors influenza viruses (WHO, 2021a). A WHO advisory group of experts reviews the influenza surveillance data generated by GISRS at biannual meetings to decide whether the seasonal influenza vaccine composition requires updating. Annual seasonal influenza vaccines are based on these surveillance data, and given the limited time available to manufacture vaccines for worldwide distribution, timely development is crucial (Hay and McCauley, 2018).

The WHO GISRS surveillance system ensures that virus strains that are prevalent during the previous season and likely to cause disease in the following season are known. Virus samples are collected and analyzed year-round by the WHO Collaborating Centers (located in Atlanta, Beijing, London, Melbourne, and Tokyo) (CDC, 2019e; WHO, 2013). Based on the antigenic and genetic characterization, antigenic cartography and predictive modeling, WHO recommends candidate viruses for the composition of the seasonal vaccines. This is done twice per year to account for seasonal influenza in the Northern and Southern Hemispheres (Ziegler et al., 2018).

Seed virus strains of the candidate viruses are produced by genetic reassortment of H1N1 and H3N2 viruses. For this genetic reassortment, the genes encoding the HA and NA proteins of the recommended influenza A viruses are reassorted with the internal protein genes of influenza A/Puerto Rico/8/34 (PR8 strain) to generate high-growth reassortant viruses. The PR8 strain is adapted to growth in chicken eggs to ensure high yield and fast production of vaccines and is safe for humans (Vemula et al., 2017). For influenza B viruses, reassortant viruses or wildtype viruses are used (Ping et al., 2016). The high growth reassortant viruses are distributed to vaccine manufacturers to start the production of vaccines.

The Landscape of Influenza Vaccine Platforms

Egg-Based Vaccine Platform

About 95 percent of the licensed seasonal influenza vaccines are manufactured in embryonated chicken eggs. The trivalent inactivated vaccine (TIV) comprises three circulating influenza strains, of which two are influenza A (H3N2 and H1N1) and one influenza B. The quadrivalent inactivated vaccine (QIV) was approved by the U.S. Food and Drug Administration (FDA) in 2012 and includes an additional B strain. Both the TIV and QIV can be manufactured in three formulations: inactivated whole virus, detergent-split virus, or subunit virus. Whole virus vaccines are immunogenic but are associated with a high level of reactogenicity. The virus is inoculated in embryonated chicken eggs and allantoic fluid is harvested. The virus is then chemically inactivated using formalin or β-propiolactone, concentrated, and purified to remove any nonviral protein contamination, such as chicken ovalbumin (Gerdil, 2003). Thiomersal or formaldehyde is used as a preservative to prevent bacterial or fungal growth. Because of their reactogenicity, whole virus vaccines have been largely replaced by split and subunit vaccines, in which additional treatment with detergents or solvents has disrupted the viral lipid envelope. The resulting incomplete viral particles contain HA, NA, and matrix proteins. These vaccines have lower reactivity than the whole virus vaccines.

Vaccines developed to mimic natural mucosal infection can theoretically induce both cellular and humoral immunity (Zhou et al., 2016). Live attenuated influenza vaccines are engineered to grow below 33°C, to limit the replication in the upper respiratory tract after inhalation (White et al., 2021). An example of this type of vaccine is FluMist/Fluenz (Zhou et al., 2016). These vaccines were first developed by serial passage of the virus in eggs under suboptimal conditions to create temperature-sensitive phenotypes. These strains then formed the "master donor" strains. These donor strains are used to contribute the internal genes, except HA and NA genes, to generate new vaccine strains with the HA and NA of the circulating strains by classical reassortment in eggs or reverse genetics (see below). Additional molecular changes have been made to internal genes to attenuate the virus and confer temperature sensitivity. The idea behind this concept is that these strains can replicate in the nasal passage but not in the respiratory tract and, in that way, elicit mucosal immune responses while not causing disease (Zhou et al., 2016).

The egg-based vaccine platform has been used since the 1940s and is well established. Because of these characteristics, it is a relatively cheap method to produce vaccines. However, it does come with some limitations that affect efficacy and limit use in case there is a high demand for vaccines, such as during a pandemic (Milián and Kamen, 2015). The egg-based platform, as described, is a time-consuming process. It takes approximately 6 months to go from the selection of strains to manufacturing vaccines to worldwide distribution (Gerdil, 2003). Given the extensive timeline required to manufacture egg-based vaccines, there is only limited time for errors. Limited availability of embryonated chicken eggs is a risk factor for this process and may delay production.

Another limitation of this platform is that the egg-based system is prone to mutations in the virus strain as it adjusts to growth in eggs (Subbarao and Barr, 2019; Wu et al., 2019). This may result in a discrepancy between the strain of the vaccine and the circulating strain, limiting the effectiveness of the vaccine, which is specifically a problem for seasonal vaccines (Pushko and Tretyakova, 2020). Additionally, there is a risk of allergic reactions to any residual egg proteins in the vaccine for people with allergies to egg antigens. However, egg allergy is not a contraindication to receiving influenza vaccine in many countries (Pushko and Tretyakova, 2020).

Cell-Based Vaccine Platform

An alternative to the egg-based approach is the use of qualified cell lines for vaccine production. This technique can use reassortant viruses or can make use of reverse genetics, a procedure that uses molecular techniques to generate a specific virus phenotype (Hegde, 2015; Wong and Webby, 2013). Using plasmid-based systems, viruses can be generated from cloned cDNA (Fodor et al., 1999; Neumann et al., 1999). After amplifying specific viral RNA fragments, the RNA is cloned into plasmids containing an

RNA polymerase I promoter sequence to drive generation of viral RNA in an antisense direction. A second RNA polymerase II promoter on the same plasmid, but in sense direction, generates mRNA for transcription of viral proteins. Alternatively, viral proteins can be expressed from a second set of plasmids. These plasmids are subsequently transfected into cells and provide the cells with all the information needed to make influenza viruses. After culture of the transfected cells, viable virus is recovered from the culture supernatant. Cell lines used to produce influenza vaccines include the Vero African monkey kidney cell, Madin-Darby canine kidney (MDCK), and the human-derived cell lines (Hegde, 2015) adapted to grow in suspension. Vaccine production using cell lines has several advantages. This technique is more easily scalable than the egg-based platform, as cell lines are widely available and can be expanded quickly. An example of an MDCK-developed vaccine that has demonstrated the potential efficiencies of this approach in productivity improvements is Flucelvax (CDC, 2021). Cells can be cryopreserved and scaled up in times of high need, which is a clear advantage in urgent situations such as pandemics if the proper facilities are available (Wong and Webby, 2013). Furthermore, this platform offers ease of manipulations in manufacturing and reduces risk of allergic reactions as the vaccine does not contain any egg components (Wong and Webby, 2013). Finally, there is a lower risk of viral mutations as seen in the egg-based platform, resulting in a vaccine with higher similarity to circulating virus strains (Harding and Heaton, 2018).

There is a risk of an adventitious virus in the cells being unintentionally introduced into the manufacturing and affecting vaccine quality. Additionally, there may be intellectual property (IP) issues around the application of reverse genetics for seasonal influenza. Therefore, this method requires extensive screening, and the process might have to be intensified to obtain the required yield.

Recombinant Influenza Vaccines

Another seasonal influenza vaccine platform that does not use chicken eggs is the recombinant protein influenza vaccine system. This is a relatively novel method that makes use of a baculovirus expression vector system. Baculoviruses are DNA viruses that can infect insects and are engineered using recombinant DNA technology to replace the gene for polyhedrin with an influenza gene of interest, such as a gene encoding a specific HA (Fabre et al., 2020). Baculovirus specifically infects *Spodoptera frugiperda* ovarian cells (Felberbaum, 2015). Because of the powerful promoter gene, a high level of HA protein production can be obtained. The SF+ cells are cultured in a fermenter and infected with the baculovirus that is engineered to express selected influenza genes. The culture is maintained for 2–4 days, the supernatants are collected, and viruses are purified by centrifugation. The protein (for the vaccine) is then extracted from the virus with detergent (Cox and Hashimoto, 2011; Invitrogen Life Technologies, n.d.). This method allows rapid scaling up, speeds up the vaccine production process, and is suitable for highly pathogenic viruses, which could be essential when a pandemic hits. A limitation of this platform is that the insect cells may not modify the expressed protein posttranscriptionally the same way as mammalian cells do, which may slightly affect the proteins antigenicity (Wong and Webby, 2013). FluBlok is an FDA-approved example of a recombinant HA trivalent vaccine derived using SF+ cells (Fabre et al., 2020; Felberbaum, 2015).

Effectiveness of Seasonal Influenza Vaccines

Vaccine effectiveness (VE) ranges from 10 to 60 percent for each seasonal vaccine component but has been relatively low for A(H3N2) viruses (Paules and Fauci, 2019). In the 2017–2018 season in the United States, the overall adjusted VE was 36 percent, with only 25 percent VE for the influenza A(H3N2) virus and 42 percent for influenza B viruses (Flannery et al., 2018). Even though effectiveness is low, the U.S. CDC still recommends vaccination as it prevents some infections, hospitalizations, and deaths. In a 9-year study of seasonal influenza from 2005 to 2014, Foppa et al. (2015) estimated that more than 40,000 lives were saved by vaccination. More recently, data from the 2018–2019 influenza season indicates vaccination prevented an estimated 4.4 million illnesses and 3,500 deaths in the United States alone (Chung et al., 2020).

The prediction of which virus strains will be circulating is an imperfect process. Therefore, vaccine strains do not always match the circulating strains, limiting VE. The egg-based vaccine platform has the additional limitation that it may result in changes in the viral genome owing to adaptation of the virus to grow in eggs (Ping et al., 2015). Additionally, there are VE challenges in specific high-risk populations, such as the elderly, owing to immunosenescence (Smetana et al., 2018), and in immunocompromised persons (Beck et al., 2012).

Repeat Immunization Effects: The Effect of Immune History or Imprinting

Another reason for the limited responses to seasonal influenza vaccination is immune history. Antibodies elicited by vaccination tend to decay within a year, in particular in older adults (Young et al., 2017). Because of antigenic drift, repeated annual administration of vaccines are required to keep up with changes in the virus. Despite extensive efforts to update vaccine strains to correct for antigenic drift, VE has been poor, particularly against H3N2 viruses (Allen and Ross, 2021).

Prior immunization can modify the VE of influenza vaccines. As part of the "antigenic sin" hypothesis, two observations are of importance: (1) antibody titers are highest to strains encountered in early childhood, and (2) vaccine antibody responses are dominated by major antigens of viruses encountered in primary childhood infections (Francis, 1960). It was originally hypothesized that people produce antibodies directed against strains encountered during early childhood at the expense of the response toward the current strain (Davenport et al., 1953). However, this hypothesis has been modified, and it is now thought that an encounter of a new influenza virus strain back-boosts titers against previously encountered strains; thus, back-boosting diminishes with antigenic distance from the new strain (Fonville et al., 2014; Lessler et al., 2012). This indicates that memory B cells induced by prior infections are activated by vaccination (Palm and Henry, 2019). Annual vaccination may accelerate this antibody refocusing on previously encountered epitopes, resulting in memory responses that do not neutralize the current strain. However, prior infection does boost the immune response and infection results in a broader antibody range than vaccination (Dugan et al., 2020). Therefore, the antibody-focusing hypothesis was developed suggesting that previously induced B cells dominate and focus the response to highly conserved epitopes between prior and prevailing vaccine strains, limiting protection when the epitope changes (Cobey and Hensley, 2017).

Correlates of Protection

The primary correlate of protection in use for seasonal influenza vaccines are hemagglutination inhibition (HI) antibody titers. HI antibodies are directed against the HA that binds sialic acid on human cells, including red blood cells, resulting in agglutination of red blood cells in solution. In the HI assay, this mechanism is used to determine whether antibodies block this cross-linking and inhibit hemagglutination (CDC, 2019d). HI antibodies are a surrogate for virus neutralization, because antibodies that block sialic acid binding inhibit the ability of the virus to infect cells (Kaufmann et al., 2017). HI antibody titers are widely used and are accepted by regulators as a correlate of protection for inactivated influenza vaccines, given that this surrogate is reasonably likely to provide clinical benefit.

However, the HI assay does not measure antibodies directed against the HA stem or other viral proteins, nor can it detect T cell responses. Therefore, this assay is not suitable for any of the universal or broadly protective vaccine candidates. In addition, the HI assay is an indirect measure, and the assay is a less sensitive measure that can be inconsistent. Therefore, innovation in measuring antibodies to HA is needed.

Universal Vaccine Development

Given the antigenic drift of influenza viruses and limitations with regard to long-lasting antibody response, there is a need to provide seasonal vaccines every year. Targeting the more conserved regions of the virus and improving vaccine-induced immunity could potentially mitigate these issues. Additionally, such strategies could be used to develop pandemic vaccines, decreasing the time it takes to produce vaccines in the traditional way. There are multiple targets of interest for the development of such universal or broadly effective vaccines.

The influenza virus requires the HA glycoprotein to attach to sialic acid-containing proteins on human cells and for the fusion between viral and endosome membranes to release viral RNA into the cell's cytoplasm (Krammer et al., 2018a). Given the importance of HA for the virulence of the virus, the HA protein is the main target for vaccines. There are two main groups of HA: group 1 and group 2, and antibodies mostly cross-react within groups (group 1: H1, H2, H5, H6, H8, H9, H11, H12, H13, H16, H17, H18; and group 2: H3, H4, H7, H10, H14, H15). Seasonal vaccines target the head domain of the HA protein that easily mutates. The HA stem and certain head regions are less prone to mutations, and antibodies toward them can potentially provide broader protection as they could neutralize various subtypes. However, these regions elicit limited immune responses (Estrada and Schultz-Cherry, 2019). Therefore, new vaccination strategies are required to target these regions. Vaccination using chimeric HA is one such option. In this strategy, the immunodominant head domain of seasonal vaccines is replaced with an avian head domain, to which humans are naïve (Nachbagauer et al., 2021). Multiple vaccinations with different heads and the same stem can elicit an immune response to targets that remain consistent, in this case, stem epitopes. An alternative to this approach replaces not the whole head, but only certain antigenic sites in the head domain to stimulate immune responses toward the conserved regions of the head. This strategy is called the mosaic HA vaccine. The Computational Optimized Broadly Reactive Antigens (COBRA) approach uses multiple HA sequences of a specific subtype to elicit broad cross-reactive responses toward the HA head and stem (Giles and Ross, 2011). The mini HA antigen vaccination approach uses epitopes only expressed on the HA stem that are structurally engineered to produce a stable construct. Repeated vaccination with these antigens can boost humoral responses toward the HA stem. Another option is the use of nanoparticle immunogens containing multiple HA glycoprotein trimers designed computationally and constructed in a controlled way so that the four HAs of licensed quadrivalent influenza vaccines are included. These "mosaic" nanoparticle immunogens have recently been shown to elicit antibody responses in preclinical models against heterologous viruses by targeting the conserved HA stem (Boyoglu-Barnum et al., 2021).

NA is a glycoprotein expressed on the surface of the virus and infected cells. The virus uses this enzyme to release the virion from infected cells. Human anti-NA antibodies can be highly and broadly protective as these inhibit the enzymatic activity of NA. NA drifts slower than HA and is well conserved within each subtype (Westgeest et al., 2012). NA content is currently not standardized in commercial vaccines, but NA inhibition has been shown to be a correlate of protection in both animal studies (Chen et al., 2018; Krammer et al., 2018b) and human studies (Maier et al., 2020; Memoli et al., 2016; Monto et al., 2015). Recombinant NA vaccines can be produced in a similar fashion as recombinant HA vaccines, with the potential to supplement current seasonal vaccines by targeting NA specifically, although there might be challenges regarding NA stability.

Internal proteins of the influenza virus are also of interest to target with vaccination strategies. The nucleoprotein and polymerase subunits are highly conserved; however, these proteins are not easily accessible for antibodies. Infected cells produce high levels of these proteins and present the antigens on major histocompatibility complex molecules, which may elicit cellular immune responses. Therefore, these proteins are investigated as potential targets for T cell-based vaccines (Carragher et al., 2008). This could be achieved using vector-based, nucleic acid, and recombinant protein vaccines.

The M2e ectodomain is a viral ion channel with limited expression on the virion but is also expressed on the cell surface of infected cells at relatively high density. The M2 protein is primarily expressed in the transmembrane and intracellular regions. However, the M2e ectodomain consists of 23 amino acids on the N terminus and is highly conserved, making it a target of interest (Saelens, 2019). Vaccines targeting M2e can induce infection-permissive (not sterilizing) immunity. In small animal models it generally protects well against infection but may permit some virus replication and morbidity.

Increasing Immunogenicity and Duration of Immune Response

To improve the current seasonal vaccines, manufacturers have aimed to improve the immunogenicity of vaccines by producing high-dose formulations of the vaccines. These higher dose formulations have been shown to improve the immunogenicity (high-dose Fluzone and Flublok) (Cox et al., 2015). Additionally, adjuvants can elicit more robust immune responses, as has been shown in the vaccine Fluad, which uses an oil-in-water adjuvant

(Tregoning et al., 2018). The research into increasing the immunogenicity has largely focused on the older population who experience immunosenescence, and current research is investigating the benefit of these dose and adjuvants changes in children with an immature immune system. Novel vaccine platforms such as DNA, RNA, and vector virus vaccines may be able to deliver high doses of antigen or provide adjuvant properties to vaccines, potentially improving immunogenicity. Additionally, vaccines developed with these platforms have the potential to induce not only antibody responses, but also $CD8^{+}$ T cell responses, potentially improving VE. However, whether these platforms indeed improve the immunogenicity for influenza vaccines remains to be investigated.

Vaccine Development in the Context of the COVID-19 Pandemic

After the WHO Country Office in China was notified of cases of pneumonia with unknown cause in Wuhan, China, on December 31, 2019 (WHO, 2020a), it took less than 2 weeks before the first genome sequence of the new coronavirus was made public on January 10, 2020 (Paden et al., 2020). The virus was later named SARS-CoV-2, and infection causes coronavirus disease 2019 (COVID-19). Two months after the sequence was first published, WHO declared COVID-19 a pandemic (WHO, 2020b). Based on previous work on SARS and MERS, the spike protein of the virus was detected as a target for vaccines, and development started after the publishing of the sequence. Even though previous research played a vital role in allowing the quick development of vaccines, the lack of funding in between the SARS and the COVID-19 pandemics slowed down the speed of development of vaccine candidates.

Vaccines were developed based on novel vaccine platforms, a development that rested on many years of basic science research (see Figure 1-3). The first phase I/II trials for vaccines used the mRNA vaccine platform and were conducted by Moderna and Pfizer-BioNTech, starting on March 16, 2020 (Moderna, 2020a) and April 23, 2020, respectively (Pfizer, 2020b). The first phase III clinical trial results were announced in November (Pfizer, 2020a) and December 2020 (Moderna, 2020b), after which Emergency Use Authorization (EUA) was provided for multiple vaccines (FDA, 2021b,c). On February 27, 2021, FDA issued EUA for a third vaccine, a one-shot regimen produced by Johnson & Johnson (Janssen) using a replication-deficient viral vector platform (FDA, 2021a). Other COVID-19 vaccines are in development and in use, and the development of various platforms has sped up vaccine development and created a greater global capacity to manufacture the many doses needed in a pandemic. Vaccine rollout over the world is currently ongoing, with more EUA of vaccine candidates to be expected in the upcoming months.

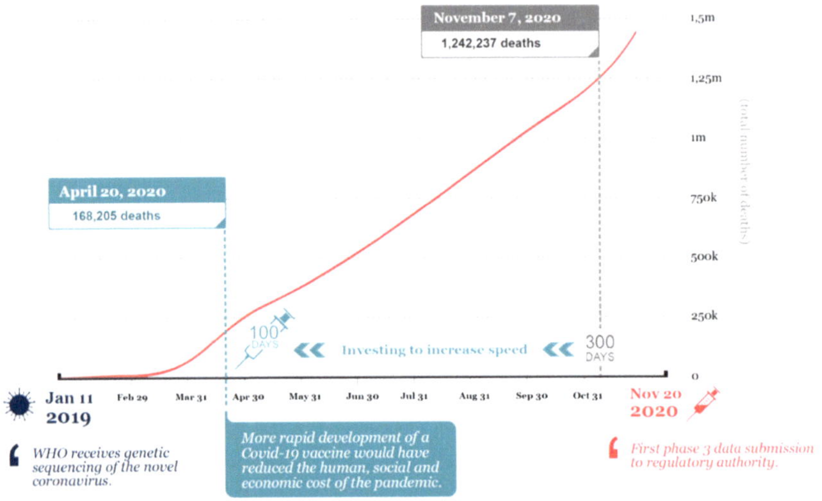

FIGURE 1-3 The COVID-19 vaccine development timeline.
NOTE: It took about 300 days from virus characterization to submission of phase III data.
SOURCE: Saville, 2021.

ORGANIZATION OF THE REPORT

The remaining chapters of this report present the committee's findings regarding the four dimensions of vaccine R&D outlined above: basic and translational science (Chapter 2), clinical science (Chapter 3), manufacturing science (Chapter 4), and regulatory science (Chapter 5). Each of these chapters ends with the committee's recommendations, informed by those findings, for applying lessons learned from the development of vaccines for COVID-19 to advance research, development, and manufacturing of vaccines for both pandemic and seasonal influenza within the respective dimension.

REFERENCES

Allen, J. D., and T. M. Ross. 2021. Next generation methodology for updating HA vaccines against emerging human seasonal influenza A(H3N2) viruses. *Scientific Reports* 11(1):4554. https://doi.org/10.1038/s41598-020-79590-7.

Beck, C. R., B. C. McKenzie, A. B. Hashim, R. C. Harris, University of Nottingham Influenza and the ImmunoCompromised Study Group, and Jonathan S. Nguyen-Van-Tam. 2012. Influenza vaccination for immunocompromised patients: Systematic review and meta-analysis by etiology. *Journal of Infectious Diseases* 206(8):1250–1259. https://doi.org/10.1093/infdis/jis487.

Boyoglu-Barnum, S., D. Ellis, R. A. Gillespie, G. B. Hutchinson, Y. J. Park, S. M. Moin, O. J. Acton, R. Ravichandran, M. Murphy, D. Pettie, N. Matheson, L. Carter, A. Creanga, M. J. Watson, S. Kephart, S. Ataca, J. R. Vaile, G. Ueda, M. C. Crank, L. Stewart, K. K. Lee, M. Guttman, D. Baker, J. R. Mascola, D. Veesler, B. S. Graham, N. P. King, and M. Kanekiyo. 2021. Quadrivalent influenza nanoparticle vaccines induce broad protection. *Nature* 592(7855):623–628. https://doi.org/10.1038/s41586-021-03365-x.

Carragher, D. M., D. A. Kaminski, A. Moquin, L. Hartson, and T. D. Randall. 2008. A novel role for non-neutralizing antibodies against nucleoprotein in facilitating resistance to influenza virus. *Journal of Immunology (Baltimore, MD: 1950)* 181(6):4168–4176. https://doi.org/10.4049/jimmunol.181.6.4168.

Carrat, F., E. Vergu, N. M. Ferguson, M. Lemaitre, S. Cauchemez, S. Leach, and A. J. Valleron. 2008. Time lines of infection and disease in human influenza: A review of volunteer challenge studies. *American Journal of Epidemiology* 167(7):775–785. https://doi.org/10.1093/aje/kwm375. https://www.ncbi.nlm.nih.gov/pubmed/18230677.

CDC (U.S. Centers for Disease Control and Prevention). 2009. Swine influenza A (H1N1) infection in two children—Southern California, March–April 2009. *Morbidity and Mortality Weekly Report* 58(15):400–402.

CDC. 2019a. *Types of influenza viruses.* https://www.cdc.gov/flu/about/viruses/types.htm (accessed October 20, 2021).

CDC. 2019b. *1968 pandemic (H3N2 virus).* https://www.cdc.gov/flu/pandemic–resources/1968-pandemic.html (accessed October 20, 2021).

CDC. 2019c. *2009 H1N1 pandemic timeline.* https://www.cdc.gov/flu/pandemic-resources/2009-pandemic-timeline.html (accessed October 20, 2021).

CDC. 2019d. *Antigenic characterization.* https://www.cdc.gov/flu/about/professionals/antigenic.htm?CDC_AA_refVal=https%3A%2F%2Fwww.cdc.gov%2Fflu%2Fprofessionals%2Flaboratory%2Fantigenic.htm (accessed October 20, 2021).

CDC. 2019e. *CDC's World Health Organization (WHO) Collaborating Center for Surveillance, Epidemiology and Control of Influenza.* https://www.cdc.gov/flu/weekly/who-collaboration.htm (accessed October 20, 2021).

CDC. 2021. *Cell-based flu vaccines.* https://www.cdc.gov/flu/prevent/cell-based.htm (accessed October 20, 2021).

Chen, Y. -Q., T. J. Wohlbold, N. -Y. Zheng, M. Huang, Y. Huang, K. E. Neu, J. Lee, H. Wan, K. Thatcher Rojas, E. Kirkpatrick, C. Henry, A.-K. E. Palm, C. T. Stamper, L. Yu-Ling Lan, D. J. Topham, J. Treanor, J. Wrammert, R. Ahmed, M. C. Eichelberger, G. Georgiou, F. Krammer, and P. C. Wilson. 2018. Influenza infection in humans induces broadly cross-reactive and protective neuraminidase-reactive antibodies. *Cell* 173(2):417–429. https://www.sciencedirect.com/science/article/pii/S0092867418303106 (accessed October 20, 2021).

Chung, J. R., M. A. Rolfes, B. Flannery, P. Prasad, A. O'Halloran, S. Garg, A. M. Fry, J. A. Singleton, M. Patel, C. Reed, U.S. Influenza Vaccine Effectiveness Network, Influenza Hospitalization Surveillance Network, and the Assessment Branch, Immunizations Services Division, Centers for Disease Control and Prevention. 2020. Effects of influenza vaccination in the United States during the 2018–2019 influenza season. *Clinical Infectious Diseases* 71(8):e368–e376.

Cobey, S., and S. E. Hensley. 2017. Immune history and influenza virus susceptibility. *Current Opinion in Virology* 22:105–111. https://doi.org/10.1016/j.coviro.2016.12.004.

Cox, M. M., and Y. Hashimoto. 2011. A fast track influenza virus vaccine produced in insect cells. *Journal of Invertebrate Pathology* 107(Suppl):S31–S41. https://doi.org/10.1016/j.jip.2011.05.003.

Cox, M. M. J., R. Izikson, P. Post, and L. Dunkle. 2015. Safety, efficacy, and immunogenicity of Flublok in the prevention of seasonal influenza in adults. *Therapeutic Advances in Vaccines* 3(4):97–108.

Davenport, F. M., A. V. Hennessy, and T. Francis, Jr. 1953. Epidemiologic and immunologic significance of age distribution of antibody to antigenic variants of influenza virus. *Journal of Experimental Medicine* 98(6):641–656. https://doi.org/10.1084/jem.98.6.641.

Drake, J. W. 1993. Rates of spontaneous mutation among RNA viruses. *Proceedings of the National Academy of Sciences* 90(9):4171–4175. https://doi.org/10.1073/pnas.90.9.4171.

Dugan, H. L., J. J. Guthmiller, P. Arevalo, M. Huang, Y.-Q. Chen, K. E. Neu, C. Henry, N.-Y. Zheng, L. Y.-L. Lan, M. E. Tepora, O. Stovicek, D. Bitar, A.-K. E. Palm, C. T. Stamper, S. Changrob, H. A. Utset, L. Coughlan, F. Krammer, S. Cobey, and P. C. Wilson. 2020. Preexisting immunity shapes distinct antibody landscapes after influenza virus infection and vaccination in humans. *Science and Translational Medicine* 12(573):eabd3601. https://doi.org/10.1126/scitranslmed.abd3601.

Estrada, L. D., and S. Schultz-Cherry. 2019. Development of a universal influenza vaccine. *Journal of Immunology* 202(2):392–398. https://doi.org/10.4049/jimmunol.1801054.

Fabre, M. L., P. N. Arrías, T. Masson, M. L. Pidre, and V. Romanowski. 2020. Baculovirus-derived vectors for immunization and therapeutic applications. *Emerging and Reemerging Viral Pathogens* 197–224. https://doi.org/10.1016/B978-0-12-814966-9.00011-1.

FDA (U.S. Food and Drug Administration). 2021a. *Janssen COVID-19 vaccine.* https://www.fda.gov/emergency-preparedness-and-response/coronavirus-disease-2019-covid-19/janssen-covid-19-vaccine.

FDA. 2021b. *Moderna COVID-19 vaccine.* https://www.fda.gov/emergency-preparedness-and-response/coronavirus-disease-2019-covid-19/moderna-covid-19-vaccine#:~:text=The%20emergency%20use%20authorization%20allows,of%20age%20and%20older (accessed October 20, 2021).

FDA. 2021c. *Pfizer-BioNTech COVID-19 vaccine.* https://www.fda.gov/emergency-preparedness-and-response/coronavirus-disease-2019-covid-19/pfizer-biontech-covid-19-vaccine (accessed October 20, 2021).

Felberbaum, R. S. 2015. The baculovirus expression vector system: A commercial manufacturing platform for viral vaccines and gene therapy vectors. *Biotechnology Journal* 10(5):702–714. https://doi.org/10.1002/biot.201400438.

Flannery, B., J. R. Chung, E. A. Belongia, H. Q. McLean, M. Gaglani, K. Murthy, R. K. Zimmerman, M. P. Nowalk, M. L. Jackson, L. A. Jackson, A. S. Monto, E. T. Martin, A. Foust, W. Sessions, L. Berman, J. R. Barnes, S. Spencer, and A. M. Fry. 2018. Interim estimates of 2017–18 seasonal influenza vaccine effectiveness - United States, February 2018. *Morbidity and Mortality Weekly Report* 67(6):180–185. https://doi.org/10.15585/mmwr.mm6706a2.

Fodor, E., L. Devenish, O. G. Engelhardt, P. Palese, G. G. Brownlee, and A. García-Sastre. 1999. Rescue of influenza A virus from recombinant DNA. *Journal of Virology* 73(11):9679–9682. https://doi.org/10.1128/JVI.73.11.9679-9682.1999.

Fonville, J. M., S. H. Wilks, S. L. James, A. Fox, M. Ventresca, M. Aban, L. Xue, T. C. Jones, N. M. H. Le, Q. T. Pham, N. D. Tran, Y. Wong, A. Mosterin, L. C. Katzelnick, D. Labonte, T. T. Le, G. van der Net, E. Skepner, C. A. Russell, T. D. Kaplan, G. F. Rimmelzwaan, N. Masurel, J. C. de Jong, A. Palache, W. E. P. Beyer, Q. M. Le, T. H. Nguyen, H. F. L. Wertheim, A. C. Hurt, A. D. M. E. Osterhaus, I. G. Barr, R. A. M. Fouchier, P. W. Horby, and D. J. Smith. 2014. Antibody landscapes after influenza virus infection or vaccination. *Science (New York, N.Y.)* 346(6212):996–1000. https://doi.org/10.1126/science.1256427.

Foppa, I. M., P. Y. Cheng, S. B. Reynolds, D. K. Shay, C. Carias, J. S. Bresee, I. K. Kim, M. Gambhir, and A. M. Fry. 2015. Deaths averted by influenza vaccination in the U.S. during the seasons 2005/06 through 2013/14. *Vaccine* 33(26):3003–3009.

Francis, T. 1960. On the doctrine of original antigenic sin. *Proceedings of the American Philosophical Society* 104(6):572–578. http://www.jstor.org/stable/985534 (accessed October 20, 2021).

Gerdil, C. 2003. The annual production cycle for influenza vaccine. *Vaccine* 21(16):1776–1779. https://doi.org/10.1016/s0264-410x(03)00071-9.

Ghebrehewet, S., P. MacPherson, and A. Ho. 2016. Influenza. *BMJ* 355:i6258. https://doi.org/10.1136/bmj.i6258.

Giles, B. M., and T. M. Ross. 2011. A computationally optimized broadly reactive antigen (COBRA) based H5N1 VLP vaccine elicits broadly reactive antibodies in mice and ferrets. *Vaccine* 29(16):3043–3054. https://doi.org/10.1016/j.vaccine.2011.01.100.

Gómez-Puertas, P., C. Albo, E. Pérez-Pastrana, A. Vivo, and A. Portela. 2000. Influenza virus matrix protein is the major driving force in virus budding. *Journal of Virology* 74(24):11538–11547. https://doi.org/10.1128/jvi.74.24.11538-11547.2000.

Harding, A. T., and N. S. Heaton. 2018. Efforts to improve the seasonal influenza vaccine. *Vaccines* 6(2):19. https://doi.org/10.3390/vaccines6020019.

Hay, A. J., and J. W. McCauley. 2018. The WHO global influenza surveillance and response system (GISRS)—A future perspective. *Influenza and Other Respiratory Viruses* 12(5):551–557. https://doi.org/10.1111/irv.12565.

Hegde, N. R. 2015. Cell culture-based influenza vaccines: A necessary and indispensable investment for the future. *Human Vaccines & Immunotherapeutics* 11(5):1223–1234. https://doi.org/10.1080/21645515.2015.1016666.

HHS (U.S. Department of Health and Human Services). 2020. *National Influenza Vaccine Modernization Strategy 2020-2030.* https://www.phe.gov/Preparedness/planning/nivms/Documents/nivms-2020-2030.pdf (accessed October 20, 2021).

Hsieh, Y.-H., S. Ma, J. X. V. Hernandez, V. J. Lee, and W. Y. Lim. 2011. Early outbreak of 2009 influenza A (H1N1) in Mexico prior to identification of pH1N1 virus. *PLOS ONE* 6(8):e23853. https://doi.org/10.1371/journal.pone.0023853.

Invitrogen Life Technologies. n.d. *Guide to baculovirus expression vector systems (BEVS) and insect cell culture techniques.* https://tools.thermofisher.com/content/sfs/manuals/bevtest.pdf (accessed October 20, 2021).

Iuliano, A. D., K. M. Roguski, H. H. Chang, D. J. Muscatello, R. Palekar, S. Tempia, C. Cohen, J. M. Gran, D. Schanzer, B. J. Cowling, P. Wu, J. Kyncl, L. W. Ang, M. Park, M. Redlberger-Fritz, H. Yu, L. Espenhaim, A. Krishnan, G. Emukule, L. van Asten, S. P. da Silva, S. Aungkulanon, U. Buchholz, M.-A. Widdowson, and J. S. Bresee for the Global Seasonal Influenza-Associated Mortality Collaborator Network. 2018. Estimates of global seasonal influenza-associated respiratory mortality: A modelling study. *Lancet* 391(10127):1285–1300. https://doi.org/10.1016/S0140-6736(17)33293-2.

Jameson, J., J. Cruz, M. Terajima, and F. A. Ennis. 1999. Human CD8+ and CD4+ T lymphocyte memory to influenza A viruses of swine and avian species. *Journal of Immunology* 162(12):7578–7583. https://www.jimmunol.org/content/jimmunol/162/12/7578.full.pdf (accessed October 20, 2021).

Janway, C. A., P. Travers, Jr., M. Walport, and M. J. Shlomchik. 2001. *Immunobiology: The Immune System in Health and Disease.* 5th ed. New York: Garland Science.

Jha, B. K., R. Pandit, R. Jha, and K. D. Manandhar. 2020. Overview of seasonal influenza and recommended vaccine during the 2016/2017 season in Nepal. *Heliyon* 6(1):e03304. https://doi.org/10.1016/j.heliyon.2020.e03304.

Johnson, N. P. A. S., and J. Mueller. 2002. Updating the accounts: Global mortality of the 1918–1920 Spanish influenza pandemic. *Bulletin of the History of Medicine* 76(1):105–115. http://www.jstor.org/stable/44446153 (accessed October 20, 2021).

Kaufmann, L., M. Syedbasha, D. Vogt, Y. Hollenstein, J. Hartmann, J. E. Linnik, and A. Egli. 2017. An optimized hemagglutination inhibition (HI) assay to quantify influenza-specific antibody titers. *Journal of Visualized Experiments* (130):55833. https://doi.org/10.3791/55833.

Kawaoka, Y., S. Krauss, and R. G. Webster. 1989. Avian-to-human transmission of the *pb1* gene of influenza A viruses in the 1957 and 1968 pandemics. *Journal of Virology* 63(11):4603–4608.

Kinsella, C. M., P. D. Santos, I. Postigo-Hidalgo, A. Folgueiras-González, T. C. Passchier, K. P Szillat, J. O. Akello, B. Álvarez-Rodríguez, and J. Martí-Carreras. 2020. Preparedness needs research: How fundamental science and international collaboration accelerated the response to COVID-19. *PLOS Pathogens* 16(10):e1008902. https://www.ncbi.nlm.nih.gov/pmc/articles/PMC7546461/pdf/ppat.1008902.pdf (accessed October 20, 2021).

Krammer, F., G. J. D. Smith, R. A. M. Fouchier, M. Peiris, K. Kedzierska, P. C. Doherty, P. Palese, M. L. Shaw, J. Treanor, R. G. Webster, and A. García-Sastre. 2018a. Influenza. *Nature Reviews Disease Primers* 4(1):3. https://doi.org/10.1038/s41572-018-0002-y.

Krammer, F., R. A. M. Fouchier, M. C. Eichelberger, R. J. Webby, K. Shaw-Saliba, H. Wan, P. C. Wilson, R. W. Compans, I. Skountzou, and A. S. Monto. 2018b. NAction! How can neuraminidase-based immunity contribute to better influenza virus vaccines? *mBio* 9(2):e02332-17. https://doi.org/10.1128/mBio.02332-17.

LePan, N. 2021. *Visualizing the history of pandemics*. https://www.visualcapitalist.com/history-of-pandemics-deadliest (accessed October 20, 2021).

Lessler, J., S. Riley, J. M. Read, S. Wang, H. Zhu, G. J. D. Smith, Y. Guan, C. Q. Jiang, and D. A. T. Cummings. 2012. Evidence for antigenic seniority in influenza A (H3N2) antibody responses in southern China. *PLOS Pathogens* 8(7):e1002802. https://journals.plos.org/plospathogens/article?id=10.1371/journal.ppat.1002802 (accessed October 20, 2021).

Lopez, C. E., and K. L. Legge. 2020. Influenza A virus vaccination: Immunity, protection, and recent advances toward a universal vaccine. *Vaccines* 8(3):1–23. https://doi.org/10.3390/vaccines8030434.

Luo, M. 2012. Influenza virus entry. *Advances in Experimental Medicine and Biology* 726:201–221. https://doi.org/10.1007/978-1-4614-0980-9_9.

Maier, H. E., R. Nachbagauer, G. Kuan, S. Ng, R. Lopez, N. Sanchez, D. Stadlbauer, L. Gresh, A. Schiller, A. Rajabhathor, S. Ojeda, A. F. Guglia, F. Amanat, A. Balmaseda, F. Krammer, and A. Gordon. 2020. Pre-existing antineuraminidase antibodies are associated with shortened duration of influenza A(H1N1)pdm virus shedding and illness in naturally infected adults. *Clinical Infectious Disease* 70(11):2290–2297. https://doi.org/10.1093/cid/ciz639.

Memoli, M. J., P. A. Shaw, A. Han, L. Czajkowski, S. Reed, R. Athota, T. Bristol, S. Fargis, K. Risos, J. H. Powers, R. T. Davey, J. K. Taubenberger, A. Moscona, J. Crowe, and D. Hoft. 2016. Evaluation of antihemagglutinin and antineuraminidase antibodies as correlates of protection in an influenza A/H1N1 virus healthy human challenge model. *mBio* 7(2):e00417-16. https://doi.org/doi:10.1128/mBio.00417-16.

Milián, E., and A. A. Kamen. 2015. Current and emerging cell culture manufacturing technologies for influenza vaccines. *BioMedical Research International*. https://doi.org/10.1155/2015/504831.

Moderna. 2020a. *Moderna announces first participant dosed in NIH-led phase 1 study of mRNA vaccine (mRNA-1273) against novel coronavirus*. https://investors.modernatx.com/news-releases/news-release-details/moderna-announces-first-participant-dosed-nih-led-phase-1-study (accessed October 20, 2021).

Moderna. 2020b. *Moderna announces publication of results from the pivotal phase 3 trial of the Moderna COVID-19 vaccine in the* New England Journal of Medicine. https://investors.modernatx.com/news-releases/news-release-details/moderna-announces-publication-results-pivotal-phase-3-trial (accessed October 20, 2021).

Monto, A. S., J. G. Petrie, R. T. Cross, E. Johnson, M. Liu, W. Zhong, M. Levine, J. M. Katz, and S. E. Ohmit. 2015. Antibody to influenza virus neuraminidase: An independent correlate of protection. *Journal of Infectious Diseases* 212(8):1191–1199. https://doi.org/10.1093/infdis/jiv195.

Nachbagauer, R., J. Feser, A. Naficy, D. I. Bernstein, J. Guptill, E. B. Walter, F. Berlanda-Scorza, D. Stadlbauer, P. C. Wilson, T. Aydillo, M. A. Behzadi, D. Bhavsar, C. Bliss, C. Capuano, J. M. Carreño, V. Chromikova, C. Claeys, L. Coughlan, A. W. Freyn, C. Gast, A. Javier, K. Jiang, C. Mariottini, M. McMahon, M. McNeal, A. Solórzano, S. Strohmeier, W. Sun, M. Van der Wielen, B. L. Innis, A. García-Sastre, P. Palese, and F. Krammer. 2021. A chimeric hemagglutinin-based universal influenza virus vaccine approach induces broad and long-lasting immunity in a randomized, placebo-controlled phase I trial. *Nature Medicine* 27(1):106–114. https://doi.org/10.1038/s41591-020-1118-7.

Neumann, G., T. Watanabe, H. Ito, S. Watanabe, H. Goto, P. Gao, M. Hughes, D. R. Perez, R. Donis, E. Hoffmann, G. Hobom, and Y. Kawaoka. 1999. Generation of influenza A viruses entirely from cloned cDNAs. *Proceedings of the National Academy of Sciences* 96(16):9345–9350. https://doi.org/10.1073/pnas.96.16.9345.

Ortiz, J. R., J. Hickling, R. Jones, A. Donabedian, O. G. Engelhardt, J. M. Katz, S. A. Madhi, K. M. Neuzil, G. F. Rimmelzwaan, J. Southern, D. J. Spiro, and J. Hombach. 2018. Report on eighth WHO meeting on development of influenza vaccines that induce broadly protective and long-lasting immune responses: Chicago, USA, 23–24 August 2016. *Vaccine* 36(7):932–938. https://doi.org/10.1016/j.vaccine.2017.11.061.

Paden, C. R., Y. Tao, K. Queen, J. Zhang, Y. Li, A. Uehara, and S. Tong. 2020. Rapid, sensitive, full-genome sequencing of severe acute respiratory syndrome coronavirus 2. *Emerging Infectious Diseases* 26(10):2401–2405. https://doi.org/10.3201/eid2610.201800.

Palm, A.-K. E., and C. Henry. 2019. Remembrance of things past: Long-term B cell memory after infection and vaccination. *Frontiers in Immunology* 10:1787. https://doi.org/10.3389/fimmu.2019.01787.

Paules, C. I., and A. S. Fauci. 2019. Influenza vaccines: Good, but we can do better. *The Journal of Infectious Diseases* 219(Suppl 1):S1–S4.

Paules, C., and K. Subbarao. 2017. Influenza. *Lancet* 390(10095):697–708. https://doi.org/10.1016/s0140-6736(17)30129-0.

Pfizer. 2020a. *Pfizer and BioNTech conclude phase 3 study of COVID-19 vaccine candidate, meeting all primary efficacy endpoints.* https://www.pfizer.com/news/press-release/press-release-detail/pfizer-and-biontech-conclude-phase-3-study-covid-19-vaccine (accessed October 20, 2021).

Pfizer. 2020b. *BioNTech and Pfizer announce completion of dosing for first cohort of phase 1/2 trial of COVID-19 vaccine candidates in Germany.* https://www.pfizer.com/news/press-release/press-release-detail/biontech-and-pfizer-announce-completion-dosing-first-cohort (accessed October 20, 2021).

Ping, J., T. J. S. Lopes, C. A. Nidom, E. Ghedin, C. A. Macken, A. Fitch, M. Imai, E. A. Maher, G. Neumann, and Y. Kawaoka. 2015. Development of high-yield influenza A virus vaccine viruses. *Nature Communications* 6(1):8148.

Ping, J., T. J. Lopes, G. Neumann, and Y. Kawaoka. 2016. Development of high-yield influenza B virus vaccine viruses. *Proceedings of the National Academy of Sciences* 113(51):E8296–E8305. https://doi.org/10.1073/pnas.1616530113.

Pushko, P., and I. Tretyakova. 2020. Influenza virus like particles (VLPs): Opportunities for H7N9 vaccine development. *Viruses* 12(5):518. https://search.proquest.com/scholarly-journals/influenza-virus-like-particles-vlps-opportunities/docview/2401567847/se-2?accountid=152665 (accessed October 20, 2021).

Saelens, X. 2019. The role of matrix protein 2 ectodomain in the development of universal influenza vaccines. *Journal of Infectious Diseases* 219(Suppl 1):S68–S74. https://doi.org/10.1093/infdis/jiz003.

Saville, M. 2021. *Lessons learned from COVID-19 vaccine development.* PowerPoint presentation. Oslo, Norway: Coalition for Epidemic Preparedness Innovations.

Sedova, E. S., D. N. Scherbinin, A. A. Lysenko, S. V. Alekseeva, E. A. Artemova, and M. M. Shmarov. 2019. Non-neutralizing antibodies directed at conservative influenza antigens. *Acta Naturae* 11(4):22–32. https://doi.org/10.32607/20758251-2019-11-4-22-32.

Smetana, J., R. Chlibek, J. Shaw, M. Splino, and R. Prymula. 2018. Influenza vaccination in the elderly. *Human Vaccines & Immunotherapeutics* 14(3):540–549. https://doi.org/10.1080/21645515.2017.1343226.

Subbarao, K., and I. Barr. 2019. A tale of two mutations: Beginning to understand the problems with egg-based influenza vaccines? *Cell Host & Microbe* 25(6):773–775. https://doi.org/10.1016/j.chom.2019.05.012.

Taubenberger, J. K., and D. M. Morens. 2006. 1918 Influenza: The mother of all pandemics. *Emerging Infectious Diseases* 12(1):15–22. https://doi.org/10.3201/eid1201.050979.

Taubenberger, J. K., and D. M. Morens. 2010. Influenza: The once and future pandemic. *Public Health Reports* 125(Suppl 3):16–26. https://pubmed.ncbi.nlm.nih.gov/20568566.

Tregoning, J. S., R. F. Russell, and E. Kinnear. 2018. Adjuvanted influenza vaccines. *Human Vaccines & Immunotherapeutics* 14(3):550–564.

Vemula, S. V., E. E. Sayedahmed, S. Sambhara, and S. K. Mittal. 2017. Vaccine approaches conferring cross-protection against influenza viruses. *Expert Review of Vaccines* 16(11):1141–1154. https://doi.org/10.1080/14760584.2017.1379396.

Viboud, C., L. Simonsen, R. Fuentes, J. Flores, M. A. Miller, and G. Chowell. 2016. Global mortality impact of the 1957–1959 influenza pandemic. *Journal of Infectious Disease* 213(5):738–745. https://doi.org/10.1093/infdis/jiv534.

Westgeest, K. B., M. de Graaf, M. Fourment, T. M. Bestebroer, R. van Beek, M. I. J. Spronken, J. C. de Jong, G. F. Rimmelzwaan, C. A. Russell, A. D. M. E. Osterhaus, G. J. D. Smith, D. J. Smith, and R. A. M. Fouchier. 2012. Genetic evolution of the neuraminidase of influenza A (H3N2) viruses from 1968 to 2009 and its correspondence to haemagglutinin evolution. *Journal of General Virology* 93(Pt 9):1996–2007. https://doi.org/10.1099/vir.0.043059-0.

White, C. L., K. Chiem, D. R. Perez, J. Santos, S. Cardenas Garcia, A. Nogales, and L. Martínez-Sobrido. 2021. A new master donor virus for the development of live-attenuated influenza B virus vaccines. *Viruses* 13(7):1278. https://doi.org/10.3390/v13071278.

WHO (World Health Organization). 2011. *Main operational lessons learnt from the WHO Pandemic Influenza A (H1N1) Vaccine Deployment Initiative.* Geneva, Switzerland: World Health Organization. https://www.who.int/influenza_vaccines_plan/resources/h1n1_vaccine_deployment_initiaitve_moll.pdf (accessed October 20, 2021).

WHO. 2013. *Global epidemiological surveillance standards for influenza.* https://www.who.int/influenza/resources/documents/WHO_Epidemiological_Influenza_Surveillance_Standards_2014.pdf (accessed October 20, 2021).

WHO. 2019. *Global influenza strategy 2019–2030.* Geneva, Switzerland: World Health Organization.

WHO. 2020a. *COVID-19 - China.* https://www.who.int/emergencies/disease-outbreak-news/item/2020-DON229 (accessed October 20, 2021).

WHO. 2020b. *WHO Director-General's opening remarks at the media briefing on COVID-19 - 11 March 2020.* https://www.who.int/director-general/speeches/detail/who-director-general-s-opening-remarks-at-the-media-briefing-on-covid-19---11-march-2020 (accessed October 20, 2021).

WHO. 2021a. *Global Influenza Surveillance and Response System (GISRS).* https://www.who.int/initiatives/global-influenza-surveillance-and-response-system (accessed October 20, 2021).

WHO. 2021b. *Vaccination.* World Health Organization Regional Office for Europe. https://www.euro.who.int/en/health-topics/communicable-diseases/influenza/vaccination (accessed October 20, 2021).

WHO. 2021c. *Influenza-estimating burden of disease*. https://www.euro.who.int/en/health-topics/communicable-diseases/influenza/seasonal-influenza/burden-of-influenza (accessed October 20, 2021).

Wong, S.-S., and R. J. Webby. 2013. Traditional and new influenza vaccines. *Clinical Microbiology Reviews* 26(3):476–492. https://doi.org/10.1128/CMR.00097-12.

Wu, N. C., L. Huibin, A. J. Thompson, D. C. Wu, W. W. S. Ng, R. U. Kadam, C.-W. Lin, C. M. Nycholat, R. McBride, W. Liang, J. C. Paulson, C. K. P. Mok, and I. A. Wilson. 2019. Preventing an antigenically disruptive mutation in egg-based H3N2 seasonal influenza vaccines by mutational incompatibility. *Cell Host & Microbe* 25(6):836–844. https://doi.org/10.1016/j.chom.2019.04.013.

Yan, S., D. Weycker, and S. Sokolowski. 2017. US healthcare costs attributable to type A and type B influenza. *Human Vaccines and Immunotherapy* 13(9):2041–2047. https://doi.org/10.1080/21645515.2017.1345400.

Young, B., X. Zhao, A. R. Cook, C. M. Parry, A. Wilder-Smith, and M. Chen I-Cheng. 2017. Do antibody responses to the influenza vaccine persist year-round in the elderly? A systematic review and meta-analysis. *Vaccine* 35(2):212–221.

Zhou, B., V. A. Meliopoulos, W. Wang, X. Lin, K. M. Stucker, R. A. Halpin, T. B. Stockwell, S. Schultz-Cherry, and D. E. Wentworth. 2016. Reversion of cold-adapted live attenuated influenza vaccine into a pathogenic virus. *Journal of Virology* 90(19):8454–8463. https://doi.org/10.1128/JVI.00163-16.

Zhu, W., C. Dong, L. Wei, and B. Z. Wang. 2021. Promising adjuvants and platforms for influenza vaccine development. *Pharmaceutics* 13(1):68. https://doi.org/10.3390/pharmaceutics13010068.

Ziegler, T., A. Mamahit, and N. J. Cox. 2018. 65 years of influenza surveillance by a World Health Organization-coordinated global network. *Influenza and Other Respiratory Viruses* 12(5):558–565. https://doi.org/10.1111/irv.12570.

2

Basic and Translational Science

This chapter addresses the first of the four dimensions of vaccine research, development, and manufacturing examined by the committee. Key findings about vaccine research and development (R&D) from COVID-19 in relation to each of these dimensions is presented in Box 2-1. It begins by describing the development of COVID-19 vaccines and then surveys the current landscape of influenza vaccines, expanding on the overview in Chapter 1. The third section considers how lessons learned from the devel-

BOX 2-1
Basic and Translational Science: Lessons Learned from the COVID-19 Pandemic

- Previous investments in basic research were essential for rapid COVID-19 vaccine development.
- Existing centers of excellence with established off-the-shelf protocols and know-how were able to move quickly to conduct needed research on novel vaccines for COVID-19.
- Vaccine effectiveness surveillance systems were in place to monitor vaccine efficacy.
- The development of a diverse portfolio of COVID-19 vaccine platforms was essential to boost manufacturing capacity, alleviate supply shortages, and mitigate unforeseen cost, distribution, and safety issues associated with individual platforms.

opment of COVID-19 vaccines can be applied to both seasonal and pandemic influenza vaccines in the dimension of basic and translational science. The final section presents recommendations drawn from those findings.

As discussed in Chapter 1, current seasonal and pandemic influenza vaccines are based on traditional vaccine platforms and concepts that induce strain-specific immunity. The seasonal vaccines require annual reformulation and readministration, or inclusion of a novel matched virus in case of a pandemic (Krammer and Palese, 2015). This process takes months, during which the population is vulnerable to infection. Broadly protective or universal influenza vaccines have the theoretical potential to mitigate the need for seasonal reformulation and annual vaccination and may also significantly enhance pandemic preparedness. However, major developments in this area are necessary to fulfil these purposes, and these types of vaccines are therefore not expected to sustain pandemic preparedness in the short term. In addition, implementation of seasonal influenza virus vaccination programs is not considered feasible in many low- and middle-income countries (LMICs). A broadly protective, universal, low-cost influenza virus vaccine that could be given as an initial prime–boost regimen with potential booster doses given at longer intervals would make influenza vaccines affordable to LMICs and would enhance vaccine coverage in high-income countries (HICs). Some evidence to date indicates that broadly protective vaccines may not achieve the high efficacy needed to control pandemic influenza and may therefore not be the solution to pandemic preparedness. Such vaccine candidates may need to be combined with vaccines targeting strain-specific neutralizing antibody epitopes (Wei et al., 2020; Zeigler et al., 2021). This chapter addresses priorities for basic and translational science that can help achieve these goals through sustained funding.

THE DEVELOPMENT OF COVID-19 VACCINES

Basic research fueled the development of a diverse vaccine portfolio for COVID-19, which began right after the first online publication of the viral sequence. Based on previous basic research on severe acute respiratory syndrome coronavirus (SARS-CoV) and Middle East respiratory syndrome coronavirus (MERS-CoV), targets for the vaccines were quickly identified and industry, government laboratories, and academia started development of vaccines.

Platforms Used to Develop COVID-19 Vaccines

Next to traditional vaccine platforms, novel platforms are being used successfully for COVID-19. Several vaccines were developed, each with a different efficacy, ranging from 51 to 95 percent, results that may depend on the platform, the location, and the time the clinical trials were conducted, as well as the included populations. The first authorized vaccines in many countries were the vaccines produced by Pfizer-BioNTech and Moderna, that make use of a modified mRNA platform (Gavi, 2021). The vaccines consist of modified mRNA encoding the prefusion-stabilized, full-length spike protein of SARS-CoV-2, which is encapsulated in lipid nanoparticles for delivery (Baden et al., 2020; Polack et al., 2020). Both vaccines were found to be safe in clinical trials; however, acute allergic reactions were reported after vaccine rollout to the population, with a reported 2.5–11.1 cases of anaphylaxis per million doses given (Blumenthal et al., 2021). With the spread of SARS-CoV-2 over the course of the pandemic, several variant viruses have emerged—some are designated as variants of concern and others as variants of interest (Subbarao, 2021). The levels of neutralizing antibody in the sera of vaccinated individuals to some of these variants, such as the beta and delta variants, was lower than against the vaccine strain (Stowe et al., 2021) though the vaccines are still highly effective in preventing severe illness and death, as they were designed to provide cross-protection against variants. The mRNA vaccine platform offers the flexibility to design booster vaccine candidates against such variants to improve efficacy. Both Pfizer-BioNTech and Moderna started phase I trials studying such variants of their vaccines in early 2021.

Another vaccine platform used by several manufacturers is the replication-deficient viral vector platform. AstraZeneca developed a vaccine in collaboration with the University of Oxford that uses a recombinant replication-deficient chimpanzee adenovirus (ChAdOx1) vector encoding the spike protein of SARS-CoV-2 (Voysey et al., 2021). The single-dose vaccine developed by Janssen (Johnson & Johnson) uses a recombinant, replication-incompetent adenovirus serotype 26 (Ad26) vector encoding the full-length, stabilized spike protein (Oliver et al., 2021). The Gamaleya National Research Centre for Epidemiology and Microbiology in Russia developed a heterologous recombinant adenovirus vaccine based on recombinant adenovirus type 26 and type 5 encoding the full-length spike protein of SARS-CoV-2 (Logunov et al., 2021). Finally, the vaccine developed by CanSino Biologics in China is a one-dose regimen like the Janssen vaccine, using adenovirus type 5 as the viral vector to encode the spike protein (Peshimam and Farooq, 2021).

Two candidates using a protein subunit vaccine platform are those developed by Novavax and the Vector Institute. The Novavax vaccine uses a stable, prefusion recombinant spike protein nanoparticle that is adjuvanted with Matrix-M. On June 14, 2021, Novavax released the results of its phase III trial (Novavax, 2021). Sanofi Pasteur also has a recombinant protein-based vaccine adjuvanted with GlaxoSmithKline's (GSK's) AS03 adjuvant in a phase III study that was initiated in May 2021 (Sanofi, 2021).

Finally, several vaccines based on whole inactivated virus have been developed. A vaccine produced by the Chinese company Sinopharm received authorization in China and from the World Health Organization (WHO) (Al Kaabi et al., 2021; Zimmer et al., 2021). A vaccine produced by another Chinese company, Sinovac, was authorized for use in China and by WHO (2021b). A vaccine by Bharat BioTech is authorized for use in India (Pokharel, 2021).

Initiatives to Fund COVID-19 Vaccine Development

To stimulate the development of COVID-19 vaccines, countries—individually and together in consortia—funded the development of multiple candidates. The United States launched Operation Warp Speed (OWS) in May 2020 as an initiative by the U.S. Department of Health and Human Services (HHS). This public–private partnership had the objective to deliver 300 million doses of a safe and effective vaccine for COVID-19 by January 2021 (GAO, 2021). The partnership included federal bodies and biopharmaceutical companies working on vaccines. OWS provided funding or contracts to support the development of the vaccines by Moderna (mRNA platform), AstraZeneca and the University of Oxford (replication-defective vector platform), Johnson & Johnson (Janssen, replication-defective vector), Novavax (protein adjuvanted), and GSK and Sanofi (protein adjuvanted) (Slaoui and Hepburn, 2020). Pfizer and BioNTech (mRNA platform) did not accept federal funding but contracted with OWS to secure 100 million doses for the United States (Zimmer and Thomas, 2020).

The Coalition for Epidemic Preparedness Innovations (CEPI), a global partnership including public, private, philanthropic, and civil society organizations, was launched in 2017 to develop vaccines for future pandemics. CEPI also aims to enable equitable access to the vaccines developed through the COVAX initiative, allowing early access of novel vaccines to LMICs. It has pledged investments of up to $1.2 billion in a diverse portfolio of vaccine candidates based on multiple platforms. Figure 2-1 depicts COVID-19 vaccines supported by CEPI. Furthermore, it has laid out a series of protocols to facilitate rapid clinical studies (CEPI, 2020). The European Union committed to investing €1 billion from the Horizon 2020 program for research and innovation to the Coronavirus Global Response Initiative, with €350 million available for vaccine development (European Commission, 2021). These and other generous funding initiatives and collaborations among many players facilitated the rapid development of COVID-19 vaccines.

The first vaccine, produced by Pfizer-BioNTech, was authorized 8 months after clinical trials began (Ball, 2021). COVID-19 vaccine development was rapid but not enough to prevent hundreds of millions of infections (WHO, 2021a) and thousands of deaths. Thus, it is crucial that the vaccination strategy for pandemic influenza involves both *preparedness*,

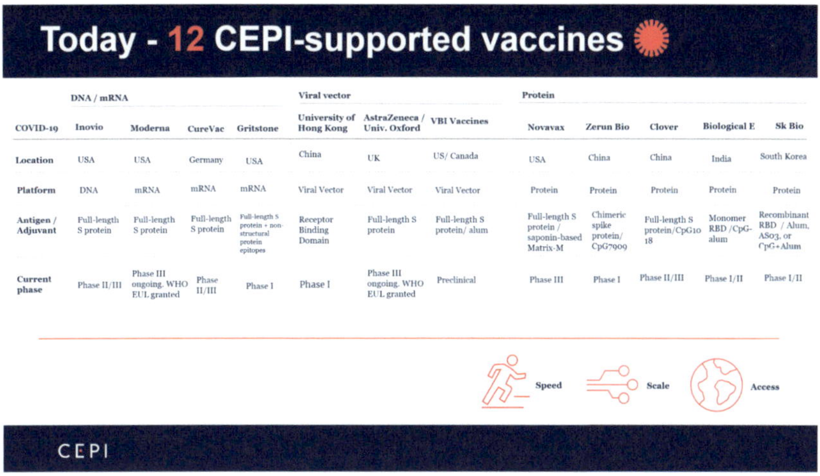

	DNA / mRNA				Viral vector			Protein				
COVID-19	**Inovio**	**Moderna**	**CureVac**	**Gritstone**	**University of Hong Kong**	**AstraZeneca / Univ. Oxford**	**VBI Vaccines**	**Novavax**	**Zerun Bio**	**Clover**	**Biological E**	**Sk Bio**
Location	USA	USA	Germany	USA	China	UK	US/ Canada	USA	China	China	India	South Korea
Platform	DNA	mRNA	mRNA	mRNA	Viral Vector	Viral Vector	Viral Vector	Protein	Protein	Protein	Protein	Protein
Antigen / Adjuvant	Full-length S protein	Full-length S protein	Full-length S protein	Full-length S protein + non-structural protein epitopes	Receptor Binding Domain	Full-length S protein	Full-length S protein/ alum	Full-length S protein / saponin-based Matrix-M	Chimeric spike protein/ CpG7909	Full-length S protein/CpG10 18	Monomer RBD /CpG-alum	Recombinant RBD / Alum, AS03, or CpG+Alum
Current phase	Phase II/III	Phase III ongoing. WHO EUL granted	Phase II/III	Phase I	Phase I	Phase III ongoing. WHO EUL granted	Preclinical	Phase III	Phase I	Phase II/III	Phase I/II	Phase I/II

FIGURE 2-1 Coalition for Epidemic Preparedness Innovations–supported COVID-19 vaccines in development.
SOURCE: Saville, 2021.

including off-the-shelf vaccines that can be strategically deployed to slow down the global spread of infection, and *response*, activating the rapid development and manufacture of highly effective vaccines.

CURRENT INFLUENZA VACCINES

Influenza vaccines have been used for more than 50 years and provide moderate protection with a vaccine effectiveness rate varying between 10 and 60 percent (Paules and Fauci, 2019). An important difference between vaccine development for COVID-19 and influenza is that trials compare the efficacy in very different populations. For COVID-19, the trials compared people not having previously been exposed to the virus or a vaccine with those that were vaccinated, while for influenza previous encounters with influenza viruses may affect the response to any tested vaccine. Therefore, given that the COVID-19 vaccines were tested in a naïve population, these vaccines could show a large effect size when comparing the vaccinated group with the non-vaccinated controls. Novel influenza vaccines, on the other hand, would be tested in populations that are likely not naïve to previous influenza exposure or even influenza vaccines. Therefore, the expected effect size for such studies would be less dramatic than those shown by COVID-19 studies. Basic research includes substantial efforts to find targets for universal or broadly effective influenza vaccines and novel correlates of protection (Corder et al., 2020). Developments in the fields of virology, vaccinology, structural biology, and immunology have contributed to improvements in pandemic preparedness and seasonal influenza vaccines. While prior influenza pandemics and worrying outbreaks of avian influenza have fueled work on influenza pandemic preparedness, the COVID-19 pandemic has resulted in a major paradigm shift in vaccine technology (Billington et al., 2020). Prior to COVID-19, mRNA platforms had been studied and defined, but there was no model for widespread adoption and distribution. In particular, the cold-chain requirements of these vaccines, especially the Pfizer vaccine requiring initial cold storage conditions of about –75°C posed a challenge for global distribution (PATH, 2020). Similarly, the sole vector-based vaccine that had been licensed for human use was an Ebola vaccine, which had limited distribution, compared to vector-based vaccines for COVID-19 (FDA, 2019). Consequently, there is much to be learned from the development, evaluation, licensing, and mass vaccination of COVID-19 vaccines for future pandemic preparedness.

Production of Seasonal Influenza Vaccines in 2021

As discussed in Chapter 1, the vast majority of the available vaccines against seasonal influenza viruses in 2021 are inactivated egg-grown vaccines, with 15.5 percent produced using cell culture platforms (Sparrow et al., 2021). For trivalent inactivated vaccines, one egg is usually needed for production of a single vaccine dose. Live attenuated influenza vaccine production has usually a higher yield as every egg can produce approximately 10 quadrivalent vaccine doses (Mohn et al., 2018). The production of pandemic vaccines in eggs takes an estimated 20–28 weeks, which poses a major time challenge. The 2009 H1N1 pandemic resulted in increased hen flocks for production of eggs for better preparedness all year, but egg production still has a long lead time. For cell culture vaccines, this timeframe can potentially be reduced to 12 weeks (Wright, 2008). However, there are proprietary obstacles associated with this technique as few cell lines have been approved and licensed (Barr et al., 2018).

Limitations of Current Seasonal Influenza Vaccines

The vaccine effectiveness (VE) of the seasonal influenza vaccine ranges from 10 to 60 percent (CDC, 2020; Paules and Fauci, 2019) (see Chapter 1). This effectiveness may be decreased because of egg-adaptive mutations that occur during production. Decreases in effectiveness may also be caused by the ongoing evolution of the circulating viruses; this can lead to a mismatch between the circulating strain and the vaccine because of the time delay between strain selection and the administration of vaccines, in particular for A(H3N2) viruses (Divino et al., 2020; The Scripps Research

Institute, 2017; Zost et al., 2017). Availability of cell-based vaccines is limited because of historical factors, with the egg-based platform having been used for decades, as well as initial higher production costs (Cox et al., 2015; Rockman et al., 2020). Few countries have adopted cell-based vaccines in large quantities despite some evidence that cell-based vaccines more closely match circulating virus strains than egg-based vaccines and may be more effective (Boikos et al., 2020; DeMarcus et al., 2019; Gouma et al., 2020; Izurieta et al., 2018; Klein et al., 2020; Krishnarajah et al., 2021; Rajaram et al., 2020a; Wang et al., 2020). As annual seasonal influenza vaccination is recommended by many countries and widespread adoption is subsidized by governments, priority is often given to the most cost-efficient vaccine if sufficiently supported by evidence, which currently relies on eggs (Friede et al., 2011). Despite this, Ruiz-Aragon et al. (2020) recently showed how using cell-based quadrivalent influenza vaccines as an alternative to egg-based vaccines is actually cost-effective and lowers burden of disease, as the higher vaccine effectiveness in cell-based vaccines put less of a strain on the health care system. In a pandemic context, these barriers may be overcome by access to reserve funding. The committee recognizes that the current manufacturing capacity, availability, and use of egg-based vaccines has held back innovation of novel platforms for influenza vaccines, particularly when contrasted with COVID-19 vaccine development.

In addition to production time, the availability of eggs is a limiting factor hindering pandemic-level vaccine production (Milián and Kamen, 2015; Ulmer et al., 2006). When a novel A(H1N1) strain emerged in 2009, seed virus production started in April, a pandemic was declared in June, and vaccines were approved in September and deployed in October (Rappuoli and Dormitzer, 2012). Despite the advantage of an established process, vaccine supply during the following 2 months was insufficient to cover target groups recommended for vaccination, as also seen for COVID-19 (IOM, 2010). Recognizing insufficient supply and vaccine nationalism, in which governments of high-income countries made deals with manufacturers to ensure distribution to their population thus inhibiting the global supply of vaccines, occurred during the 2009 influenza pandemic and COVID-19 pandemic, the committee urges the building of infrastructure for surge capacity to ensure preparedness during the next impending influenza pandemic. After further research has been conducted, WHO can evaluate on the basis of the acquired data whether widespread investment into novel vaccine platforms is warranted and advise on vaccines to be stockpiled.

Egg-based vaccine production is an engrained part of the public health response to influenza. For new vaccines to be commercially viable they have to be at least as effective as the standard of care—egg-based vaccines (Newland et al., 2021). These requirements by regulatory agencies based on confirming the presence of HI antibodies has been an impediment to development of new vaccines. There is a need to create and agree upon correlates of protection for vaccines that do not induce HI antibodies. Defining such correlates needs to be determined in the context of exposure using studies into vaccine efficacy during an outbreak. Vaccines produced using novel platforms that target the traditional antigenic targets for influenza, such as HA, can use the HI assay as a correlate of protection. However, innovations to these assays are needed to ensure they can be performed faster, cheaper, and with more consistent results.

The COVID-19 pandemic was pivotal for the evolution of mRNA vaccines, which had not been tested in large populations previously. However, preclinical research resulting from the SARS-CoV and MERS-CoV outbreaks provided the foundation for the current COVID-19 vaccines. mRNA vaccines came to the forefront during COVID-19 because they could be rapidly manufactured and deployed, and they were more immunogenic than recombinant protein vaccines (Lederer et al., 2020). Importantly, the COVID-19 pandemic provided the first opportunity to demonstrate that mRNA vaccines can be safe and highly effective, leading to licensure (Baden et al., 2020; Polack et al., 2020). A number of factors will influence whether mRNA vaccine platforms are adopted for influenza vaccine development, including relative efficacy, manufacturing capacity, and costs of manufacture and distribution.

Prior Strain Immunity and the Role of Antigenic Drift

Influenza vaccines that are currently on the market induce neutralizing antibodies against the head of the influenza virus HA protein (Krammer, 2019). Due to antigenic drift among circulating virus strains (see Chapter 1), as well as antibody decay, the protection afforded by vaccine-induced antibodies is short lived. The strains used to formulate influenza vaccines are reviewed biannually, and vaccines are readministered to keep up with changes in the viruses. Despite extensive efforts to update vaccine strains to keep pace with antigenic drift, the poor vaccine effectiveness against A(H3N2) viruses persists (Belongia et al., 2017; Rajaram et al., 2020b). As discussed above, this subtype has undergone more rapid antigenic change resulting in greater mismatch between vaccine and circulating strains (Bedford et al., 2015; Paules et al., 2017). Mutations and antigenic change can also arise upon adaptation of viruses to growth in eggs, adding to the risk that the circulating strains and the vaccine strain are different, again limiting vaccine efficacy (Hampson et al., 2017; Paules et al., 2017; Zost et al., 2017). Repeated vaccination may also contribute to poor vaccine immunogenicity (Huang et al., 2017; Leung et al., 2021; Mosterín Höpping et al., 2016; Thompson et al., 2016) and effectiveness against A(H3N2) viruses

(Belongia et al., 2017; Saito et al., 2017; Morimoto and Takeishi, 2018). Effects of influenza virus exposure history on influenza vaccine responses are complex and not well understood. It is well established that infection or vaccination with a prevailing strain will boost antibody titers against prior strain variants. This phenomenon was termed *original antigenic sin* because it was thought that the continued production of antibodies against the earliest encountered strain could be detrimental to production of antibodies against the prevailing strain (Francis, 1960). More recent studies demonstrate that titer rise is greatest against the prevailing strain and decreases with increasing antigenic distance from the prevailing strain (Fonville et al., 2014). This back-boosting of antibody titers against strains encountered earlier in life is thought to be mediated by recall of memory B cells that recognize epitopes that are conserved between prior and prevailing strains (Fonville et al., 2014; Kelvin and Zambon, 2019; Nguyen-Contant et al., 2021). Continued back-boosting of antibodies against past strains may better account for the tendency for antibody titers to be highest against early life strains than the original antigenic sin hypothesis. Similarly, memory recall is likely to account for protection associated with prior infections (Fonville et al., 2014), including infection occurring early in life. Imprinting is a phenomenon whereby protection against novel A(H5N1) and A(H7N9) viruses has been associated with birth cohort and in turn with early life infection with viruses that share protective stem epitopes (Gostic et al., 2016). Nevertheless, the substantial evidence from repeated vaccination studies also indicates that existing immunity can attenuate antibody responses to prevailing vaccine strains. The antibody focusing hypothesis has been proposed to account for differences in effects of existing immunity and in effects of repeat vaccination between seasons. This hypothesis suggests that previously induced B cells dominate and focus the response on epitopes that are conserved between prior and prevailing vaccine strains, limiting protection when the epitope changes (Cobey and Hensley, 2017; Krammer, 2019). Greater understanding of the mechanisms underlying the effects of existing immunity is vital for vaccine development.

Conclusion 2-1: A priority focus for future research on influenza vaccines is how to overcome issues associated with viral antigenic drift and annual vaccination, and the potential of novel vaccine platforms to circumvent such effects. Improved characterization of B cell responses may help to validate current theories that vaccines recall existing memory B cells but do not efficiently induce de novo B cell responses against variant epitopes in new vaccine strains. This may further guide the rational design of vaccines and adjuvants to provide broader and more durable immune responses.

The Need for Universal Influenza Vaccines

Vaccines targeting conserved epitopes of the influenza virus show promising immunogenicity. Universal influenza vaccines (UIV) theoretically have the potential to provide protection against both seasonal and pandemic strains (Arinaminpathy et al., 2020) (see Chapter 1). As influenza viruses are diverse, there are many possible ways to define "universal" coverage of a vaccine. Criteria for UIV range from the degree and duration of protection to the strains it protects against (Gottlieb and Ben-Yedidia, 2014). WHO has called for the development of a vaccine that "prevents severe disease from all forms of influenza A by 2027, which would prevent pandemics" (Eisenstein, 2019). Other institutions, such as the National Institute of Allergy and Infectious Diseases (NIAID), have developed strategic plans for developing UIVs that hold different criteria (Erbelding et al., 2018). NIAID criteria state that a universal vaccine should: (1) "be at least 75 percent effective," (2) "protect against group I and II influenza A viruses," (3) "have durable protection that lasts at least 1 year," and (4) "be suitable for all age groups" (NIAID, 2021). New technologies have become available and accessible now more than ever and could help move us to a new era of influenza vaccines. These could aid in developing vaccines that not only induce antibody responses but also $CD8^+$ cytotoxic T cell responses that may provide more long-lasting effectiveness.

There are multiple barriers to the development of UIV candidates. The main gap in the development of UIVs is the necessary clinical research (see Chapter 3). Basic research has provided a number of candidates for UIVs as well as vaccine platforms, but challenges associated with clinical development, such as regulatory and economic barriers, contribute to a bottleneck in development (Cox et al., 2015; Nachbagauer and Krammer, 2017). Many of the UIV approaches are studied in silos; being tested as individual products that may or may not lead to an effective vaccine that can protect against future drift variants. An approach would be to combine different strategies in a multivalent vaccine (e.g., head and stem HA in combination, hemagglutinin (HA) and neuraminidase (NA) UIV, internal influenza proteins plus outer glycoproteins) or heterologous prime-boost strategies. Little testing is being performed with these strategies, which have been used in other vaccine development programs, such as AIDS vaccines. To implement such plans, it would be valuable for institutions to explore these approaches via funding support and working with issues related to intellectual property to create a culture of shared goals.

Early clinical trials (phase I and II) are critical for the generation of safety and immunogenicity data required to identify promising antigens and platform constructs and to select candidates for phase III efficacy trials. These types of vaccines are unlikely to replace seasonal vaccines soon, but they could be rolled out as an early pandemic control measure that does not require prior knowledge of the pandemic strain. Additionally, ongoing research is developing ways to improve the effectiveness of seasonal vaccines, such as improved adjuvants, novel platforms, and inclusion of NA antigens. These investigations may result in influenza vaccine candidates with a broader protection (e.g. "supraseasonal," or pan-H1 or pan-H3 vaccines) than the strain-specific seasonal vaccines currently in use.

It has been suggested that the COVID-19 pandemic could have been significantly offset if there had been an off-the-shelf prepared vaccine. It is predicted that even if such an off-the-shelf vaccine had a much lower efficacy, it could have slowed the progression of the pandemic while more specific and efficacious vaccines were being developed (Graham, 2021). To respond to a pandemic, the breath of the immune response may be more critical than the durability of the response. Therefore, improvement of seasonal influenza vaccines may offer the most relevant options in the near future for pandemic response preparedness.

Conclusion 2-2: The continued development and clinical assessment of vaccines targeting conserved epitopes and improved seasonal influenza vaccines with the goal of establishing a pandemic-ready stockpile is a priority. However, the usefulness of broadly protective influenza virus vaccines/UIV is not limited to pandemic preparedness. Highly effective UIV candidates would also abolish the need for matched seasonal vaccines and thereby increase vaccine uptake globally, leading to a reduced burden of seasonal influenza on global health and decreased susceptibility of the global population against zoonotic influenza virus outbreaks or emerging pandemic influenza viruses.

BASIC AND TRANSLATIONAL SCIENCE: APPLYING LESSONS FROM THE DEVELOPMENT OF COVID-19 VACCINES TO VACCINES FOR INFLUENZA

Funding Basic Research

The committee recognizes that the long-term investments in basic research have resulted in infrastructure to support the development of seasonal, broad, and universal influenza vaccines, with novel immune correlates of protection (Lim et al., 2020; Newland et al., 2021). Previous investments in basic research were essential for rapid vaccine development; and academic and industry researchers with established off-the-shelf protocols and know-how were able to move quickly to conduct needed research on novel vaccines for COVID-19. These tools will also aid in improving influenza pandemic preparedness. Similarly, sustained and appropriate investments in basic and translational science on influenza (Erbelding et al., 2018) and earlier novel coronavirus outbreaks (Begum et al., 2020) provided an evidence base for rapid development of stabilized spike-based COVID-19 vaccines (Begum et al., 2020; Wu et al., 2021), experience which can be capitalized on for future influenza vaccine work (Erbelding et al., 2018).

During interpandemic periods, funding has generally been insufficient to build and maintain capacity for manufacture and deployment of pandemic vaccines. There were many opportunities to prepare for the emergence of more SARS-CoV-like viruses between 2002 and 2020 (Saif, 2020). However, as the SARS-CoV epidemic ended and MERS-CoV outbreaks declined, and as a consequence of the decrease in perceived likelihood of need and profitability of these vaccines, funding to maintain R&D of these vaccines was reduced (Begum et al., 2020). During an outbreak, it is typical for funding to be available for the R&D of strategies leading to a phase I study. However, as soon as the outbreak resolves, funding is decreased because funding agencies are quick to move on (GPMB, 2019). For novel influenza pandemic strains, fluctuations in funding combined with the need to wait until there is active transmission to test vaccine efficacy significantly slows vaccine development, as seen with the Ebola vaccine. To ensure vaccine preparedness for the next pandemic it is essential to interrupt this pattern of discontinuation of funding for vaccine development once case numbers decline and the likelihood for potential profit margins decreases. There is a large discrepancy between the cost of a pandemic and what it would cost to consistently fund the research required for preparedness. In a non-pandemic context, funding has been insufficient for investment in capacity building and improving the public health infrastructure, thus limiting sustainable efforts to prepare for an outbreak (NAM, 2016). A continuous source of funding is necessary to prevent patterns of spikes and deserts in the funding landscape, as the current strategy is highly ineffective. While funding vaccine research is costly, ad hoc clinical trials introduce far more financial and operational inefficiencies. For example, cost analyses show that the price of developing a new vaccine from the preclinical testing phase through phase IIA trials is up to $350 million (Gouglas et al., 2018). For perspective, total global spending on COVID-19 vaccines is projected to be as high as $157 billion through 2025 (Mishra, 2021). A World Bank report estimates that a severe pandemic such as the influenza H1N1 pandemic of 1918 could cost 5 percent of the global gross domestic product. It also estimates that the annual cost of a moderate to severe pandemic would cost $570 billion annually or 0.7 percent of global income, while funding pandemic preparedness would cost just $4.5 billion, less than $1 per person (IWG, 2017). Economic impact studies like this show how costly it is to the global economy when the world is underprepared for a pandemic.

Conclusion 2-3: Sufficient funding for continuous research in the basic science of influenza vaccines is paramount to ensuring preparedness for a pandemic outbreak. Current investments are inadequate during interpandemic periods.

Using Novel Platforms for Influenza Vaccines

The COVID-19 pandemic has been a driving force for vaccine innovation, and has shown us the value of the mRNA vaccine technology (Chu et al., 2021; Vasireddy et al., 2021). At present, mRNA vaccines are expensive, capacity to manufacture them is limited, reactogenicity is relatively high—which may limit use in young children, and it is difficult to distribute them to LMICs given the cold chain required for these vaccines (Knezevic et al., 2021; Rosa et al., 2021). However, COVID-19 mRNA vaccines were developed rapidly out of need, without time to test ways in which to improve stability. With further developments and improvements of this platform, and uptake by more manufacturers, these challenges can be overcome. For example, during the COVID-19 pandemic response, for the first time, there was an essentially seamless transition between trial phases with a single protocol (NCIRS, 2020). Accordingly, further R&D on novel platforms is suggested, including increasing the number of manufacturers in different geographic areas to overcome these challenges. Expanding the number of manufacturers globally can also aid in situations where there are shortages caused by other factors unrelated to a pandemic, such as infrastructure damage caused by natural disasters.

Recombinant protein vaccines may be a cost-effective and efficient way of producing influenza vaccines compared to the mRNA platform as they have already been shown to be safe and effective and the infrastructure for production is already in place (Dunkle and Izikson, 2016; Pollet et al., 2021). Recombinant protein vaccines, such as FluBlok, have been developed and licensed for influenza but require a dose of HA that is three times higher than that used in egg-based vaccines (Wong and Webby, 2013). Development of protein vaccines for pandemic influenza may be less challenging than for SARS-CoV-2, as different HA proteins are expressed at comparable and relatively high levels using recombinant baculovirus insect cell expression systems (Jazayeri and Poh, 2019; Krammer, 2020). While recombinant protein vaccines are relatively easy to develop and manufacture, a rate-limiting step in the development for such vaccines for pandemic influenza may be the need for adjuvants to increase immunogenicity and efficacy (Coffman et al., 2010; Pollet et al., 2021). Generally, each vaccine antigen-adjuvant combination that is developed must be licensed, rather than generic licenses for adjuvants, which poses a challenge for development of new combinations. However, research into adjuvant combinations should not be forgotten in a vaccine R&D strategy because of its relative value to optimizing vaccine efficacy and dose sparing. Preclinical toxicity studies and clinical trials are therefore required for each new combination. Continuous research is needed to understand the mechanism of action and safety of adjuvants and enhanced efforts to find more efficacious adjuvants than currently available. Additionally, there is a need for licensing and building capacity to manufacture adjuvants. This will require funding to increase preclinical and clinical trial facilities.

The differences in cost of vaccines between various older and more novel vaccine platforms (e.g., egg-based versus cell culture, mRNA, or recombinant protein based) are defined by a plethora of factors, including the materials used for the production and intellectual property. Given that some vaccine platforms (reverse genetics, mRNA, recombinant protein) are relatively new, proprietary issues may result in higher costs when aiming to expand capacity. Next to the direct costs of vaccine manufacturing, the clinical work required to determine safety and efficacy to allow the vaccines to be considered for authorization and approval is an extremely costly process that represents a high risk for industry (Plotkin et al., 2017).

Conclusion 2-4: With respect to vaccine development platforms, a priority is the development of strategies for the rational choice of platforms that balances vaccine effectiveness, speed of development, and cost as the pandemic progresses. For instance, a moderately effective vaccine might be acceptable if readily available, and it can be replaced by more effective or lower cost vaccines later.

Standardizing Assays, Reagents, and Animal Models

To strengthen and adapt the vaccine development pipeline to accommodate new vaccine platforms, standardization of assays, reagents, and animal models is essential. Allowing sufficient flexibility in the details of assay design, especially for later-stage development, is essential to allow for the refinement of assays that is needed to achieve the automation, throughput, and performance standards needed to support the large-scale clinical trials that lead to vaccine authorization or licensure. After basic research characterization of potential targets for vaccines, the first phase of vaccine development involves preclinical research, including both in vitro work and animal studies to test safety and immunogenicity. Animal studies usually involve rodents and, in later stages, ferrets and sometimes non-human primates for immunological studies (FDA, 2015). Development of new reagents, particularly for ferrets, guinea pigs, and hamsters, is necessary if vaccine assessment will be performed in these preclinical animal models. Following those studies, vaccine candidates are assessed in regulatory applications, such as the investigational new drug application to the U.S. Food and Drug Administration (FDA), before receiving approval for in-human testing. Human studies involve three main phases, followed by a postmarketing surveillance phase (FDA, 2015; Slaoui and Hepburn, 2020). Clinical trials start with phase I studies in a small group of adults to assess safety; the type and extent of the immune response may be monitored. In the absence of safety concerns, the vaccine will move to phase II studies, which are conducted in a larger group of several hundred adults and may include people from risk groups. The safety, immunogenicity, proposed dosing and dosing schedule will be determined in these studies. Finally, the vaccine candidate moves to phase III studies, which include thousands to tens of thousands of individuals, often in a double-blind, randomized, placebo-controlled study to assess safety and efficacy. Efficacy studies may determine whether the vaccine prevents infection with the virus; prevents (severe) disease, hospitalization, or death; and induces a protective immune response by assessing antibody production and other immune markers (FDA, 2015).

To achieve clinical endpoints, the prevalence of the virus in a population (attack rate) is a determinant of how many people need to be studied and for how long. Given the relatively low incidence of clinically apparent seasonal influenza, clinical trials are often large, making them costly and time consuming. This discourages pharmaceutical companies from engaging in next-generation influenza virus vaccine development. Having immune correlates of protection to assess in clinical trials would streamline the vaccine development pipeline. New vaccine platforms require their own immune correlates, and these should be assessed using standardized assays to allow for the comparison of immunogenicity and efficacy between different vaccine candidates and for decision making. For COVID-19, this was not predetermined and comparing vaccine trial results was therefore challenging. Correlates of protection that are being assessed for COVID-19 are not yet well defined, though neutralizing antibody responses to the spike protein are often used as a proxy and can be assessed by multiple assays reported as values or titers (Khoury et al., 2021; Klasse et al., 2021). Convalescent plasma was often included as a comparator; however, this was not standardized across studies. International standards were not readily available and clinical trials were developed and conducted before standards were available. This example indicates the need for research to define correlates of protection and assay standardization *before* a pandemic, given the short response time in pandemic conditions.

After the development of novel vaccines, there is a need to develop new endpoints to provide guidance to regulatory agencies, like FDA, for assessment of novel vaccines that do not induce hemagglutinin inhibition

(HI) antibodies (Lim et al., 2020; Weir and Gruber, 2016). New seasonal influenza virus strains are selected on the basis of specific hemagglutination-inhibiting (HI) antibody responses, and seasonal influenza vaccines do not require field efficacy trials each time they are updated (Weir and Gruber, 2016). When updating a vaccine containing new antigens for the seasonal influenza vaccine, manufacturers submit a supplement for their existing vaccine license. Supplements for live attenuated, but not inactivated, vaccines require a study in approximately 300 adults to demonstrate sufficient attenuation (Weir and Gruber, 2016). The current system promotes the types of vaccines already available as it uses HI antibodies as the correlate of protection for influenza. Age also affects immunity, which is not currently considered in the correlate of protection, but it should be addressed (Reber et al., 2012). Another effect of the focus on the HI assay is the lack of attention to NA in assessing VE. Traditional vaccines contain some NA, but the amount of NA in vaccines is not standardized, and NA antibodies are not measured in a standardized assay (Gomez Lorenzo and Fenton, 2013). Therefore, standardization and sole focus on one type of assay and correlates of protection might stand in the way of innovation. During the influenza season, countries such as the United States, Canada, Russia, Australia, and multiple European countries routinely use the test-negative design to estimate VE, and conduct ad hoc assessments of vaccine immunogenicity (Sullivan et al., 2014). The committee proposes investments that support research into new clinical endpoints on an ongoing basis, and that assays to assess correlates of protection are standardized for each vaccine platform.

From a technical point of view, the establishment of correlates of protection and their broad use across different vaccines, platforms, developers, and regulatory agencies would be facilitated by the use of standardized assays and reagents. For influenza, there have already been efforts to standardize protocols and establish quality assurance systems. The Standardization and Development of Assays for Assessment of Influenza Vaccine Correlates of Protection (FLUCOP) initiative was developed with the goal of standardizing assays for correlates of protection and is focused on providing protocols and training videos to make these assays available globally. Funding for FLUCOP has come from the European Union and will end in 2022 (FLUCOP, 2020). Additionally, the Consortium for the Standardization of Influenza Seroepidemiology (CONSISE) started in 2011 as a partnership of various global organizations without specific funding. CONSISE aims to standardize influenza serology worldwide, and has developed standardized research protocols for epidemiology, clinical data collection, and biological sample collection, processing, and research (CONSISE, 2021).

Conclusion 2-5: Advances in influenza vaccine development will require standardized assays, reagents, and animal models for the development of novel correlates of protection. This work should be facilitated by WHO's development of international standards for these research tools.

Global Expansion of Clinical Research

Global collaboration and distribution of know-how and reagents are essential for the development of vaccines, correlates of protection, and global clinical trial capacity (human capital). Clinical research presents a fundamental gap in the R&D of vaccines. There are several candidates for universal influenza vaccines and several new vaccine platforms, but clinical testing is a bottleneck that should be prioritized. Clinical development should be carried out on a global scale, requiring global coordination. However, as of 2021, most of the universal influenza vaccine trials are performed in the United States. At the time of print, the National Institutes of Health (NIH) reports as many as 25 clinical trials being conducted globally. Of these, 11 are in the United States, 6 in Europe, 4 in the Middle East, and 2 in North Asia (NIH, 2021). It is essential that vaccines are tested in diverse populations and, therefore, expansion of the conduction of clinical trials globally is vital.

Impediments to the necessary collaboration include resource limitations and the complexities of multi-national trials, including regulatory hurdles and incompatibility. Few countries have the capacity and expertise to perform such trials. Note that WHO has previously encouraged LMIC manufacturers to move into the influenza vaccine space, and these efforts were supported in the past by funding from the Biomedical Advanced Research Development Authority (BARDA) in the United States (Berlanda Scorza, 2017). However, there is a need for a local market to sustain influenza vaccine development. There will be a need to build appropriate facilities and train local experts, which will require political support and a local market for influenza vaccine to sustain production.

RECOMMENDATIONS

Based on the findings and conclusions presented in this chapter, the committee makes the following recommendations regarding the research, development, and manufacturing of seasonal and pandemic influenza vaccines in the dimension of basic and translational science.

Recommendation 2-1: The U.S. Department of Health and Human Services, through the National Institute of Allergy and Infectious Diseases, the Biomedical Advanced Research and Development Authority,

and the U.S. Department of Defense, as well as other corresponding governmental and funding agencies domestically and abroad, should invest, proportionate to the enormous costs of pandemics, in basic and translational research to reveal a diverse array of influenza vaccines, using different platforms, viral targets, adjuvants, and delivery systems. This will allow selection of the candidates most fit for purpose to be brought to authorization and sufficient production and distribution to optimize the control of influenza across diverse settings and phases of pandemics and epidemics.

Recommendation 2-2: The World Health Organization should advocate and coordinate with multi-lateral stakeholders (e.g., the Coalition for Epidemic Preparedness Innovations), governments, funding agencies, the vaccine industry, and philanthropic organizations to build global capacity for robust and internationally comparable preclinical, clinical, and immunological assessments of influenza vaccine candidates, including novel candidates that use innovative structures, targets, and delivery systems to potentially broaden or improve protection.

Recommendation 2-3: International research networks (e.g., the National Institutes of Health/U.S. Centers for Disease Control and Prevention funding networks) supported by governments and funding agencies, the World Health Organization, and the vaccine industry should support, carefully plan, and conduct multi-center international clinical trials and field studies to compare emerging vaccines with standard vaccines in, among others, geographically, demographically, and immunologically diverse populations to inform rational and situation-based use and manufacture of an extended array of vaccines.

Recommendation 2-4: National regulators should engage with the vaccine industry and academic researchers in the development, standardization, and implementation of innovative assays to evaluate vaccines that induce immunity through mechanisms other than strain-specific neutralizing hemagglutination-inhibiting antibodies in order to reach consensus on the validation of these assays that will allow approval or licensure of influenza vaccines based on a broader range of assays that reflect induction of immunity.

REFERENCES

Al Kaabi, N., Y. Zhang, S. Xia, Y. Yang, M. M. Al Qahtani, N. Abdulrazzaq, M. Al Nusair, M. Hassany, J. S. Jawad, J. Abdalla, S. E. Hussein, S. K. Al Mazrouei, M. Al Karam, X. Li, X. Yang, W. Wang, B. Lai, W. Chen, S. Huang, Q. Wang, T. Yang, Y. Liu, R. Ma, Z. M. Hussain, T. Khan, M. Saifuddin Fasihuddin, W. You, Z. Xie, Y. Zhao, Z. Jiang, G. Zhao, Y. Zhang, S. Mahmoud, I. ElTantawy, P. Xiao, A. Koshy, W. A. Zaher, H. Wang, K. Duan, A. Pan, and X. Yang. 2021. Effect of 2 inactivated SARS-CoV-2 vaccines on symptomatic COVID-19 infection in adults: A randomized clinical trial. *JAMA* 326(1):35–45.

Arinaminpathy, N., S. Riley, W. S. Barclay, C. Saad-Roy, and B. Grenfell. 2020. Population implications of the deployment of novel universal vaccines against epidemic and pandemic influenza. *Journal of the Royal Society Interface* 17(164):20190879.

Baden, L. R., H. M. El Sahly, B. Essink, K. Kotloff, S. Frey, R. Novak, D. Diemert, S. A. Spector, N. Rouphael, C. B. Creech, J. McGettigan, S. Khetan, N. Segall, J. Solis, A. Brosz, C. Fierro, H. Schwartz, K. Neuzil, L. Corey, P. Gilbert, H. Janes, D. Follmann, M. Marovich, J. Mascola, L. Polakowski, J. Ledgerwood, B. S. Graham, H. Bennett, R. Pajon, C. Knightly, B. Leav, W. Deng, H. Zhou, S. Han, M. Ivarsson, J. Miller, and T. Zaks. 2020. Efficacy and safety of the mRNA-1273 SARS-CoV-2 vaccine. *New England Journal of Medicine* 384(5):403–416.

Ball, P. 2021. The lightning-fast quest for COVID vaccines—and what it means for other diseases. *Nature* 589(7840):16–18.

Barr, I. G., R. O. Donis, J. M. Katz, J. W. McCauley, T. Odagiri, H. Trusheim, T. F. Tsai, and D. E. Wentworth. 2018. Cell culture-derived influenza vaccines in the severe 2017-2018 epidemic season: A step towards improved influenza vaccine effectiveness. *NPJ Vaccines* 3:44.

Bedford, T., S. Riley, I. G. Barr, S. Broor, M. Chadha, N. J. Cox, R. S. Daniels, C. P. Gunasekaran, A. C. Hurt, A. Kelso, A. Klimov, N. S. Lewis, X. Li, J. W. McCauley, T. Odagiri, V. Potdar, A. Rambaut, Y. Shu, E. Skepner, D. J. Smith, M. A. Suchard, M. Tashiro, D. Wang, X. Xu, P. Lemey, and C. A. Russell. 2015. Global circulation patterns of seasonal influenza viruses vary with antigenic drift. *Nature* 523(7559):217–220.

Begum, J., M. Nasir Akbar, K. Dev, B. Buyamayum, W. Mohd Yaqoob, and M. Raza. 2020. Challenges and prospects of COVID 19 vaccine development based on the progress made in SARS and MERS vaccine development. *Transboundary and Emerging Diseases*. August 20.

Belongia, E. A., D. M. Skowronski, H. Q. McLean, C. Chambers, M. E. Sundaram, and G. De Serres. 2017. Repeated annual influenza vaccination and vaccine effectiveness: Review of evidence. *Expert Review of Vaccines* 16(7):1–14.

Berlanda Scorza, F. 2017. Advancing new vaccines against pandemic influenza in low-resource countries. *Vaccine* 35(40):5397–5402.

Billington, J., I. Deschamps, S. C. Erck, J. L. Gerberding, E. Hanon, S. Ivol, J. W. Shiver, J. A. Spencer, and J. Van Hoof. 2020. Developing vaccines for SARS-CoV-2 and future epidemics and pandemics: Applying lessons from past outbreaks. *Health Security* 18(3):241–249.

Blumenthal, K. G., L. B. Robinson, C. A. Camargo Jr., E. S. Shenoy, A. Banerji, A. B. Landman, and P. Wickner. 2021. Acute allergic reactions to mRNA COVID-19 vaccines. *JAMA* 325(15):1562–1565.

Boikos, C., G. C. Sylvester, J. S. Sampalis, and J. A. Mansi. 2020. Relative effectiveness of the cell-cultured quadrivalent influenza vaccine compared to standard, egg-derived quadrivalent influenza vaccines in preventing influenza-like illness in 2017-2018. *Clinical Infectious Diseases* 71(10):e665–e671.

CDC (U.S. Centers for Disease Control and Prevention). 2020. *Influenza (flu) vaccine effectiveness studies*. https://www.cdc.gov/flu/vaccines-work/effectiveness-studies.htm (accessed October 19, 2021).

CEPI (Coalition for Epidemic Preparedness Innovations). 2020. *2020 annual progress report: Covering the period from 1 January–31 December*. https://cepi.net/wp-content/uploads/2021/03/CEPI-2020-Annual-Report.pdf (accessed October 19, 2021).

Chu, L., R. McPhee, W. Huang, H. Bennett, R. Pajon, B. Nestorova, B. Leav, and mRNA Study Group. 2021. A preliminary report of a randomized controlled phase 2 trial of the safety and immunogenicity of mRNA-1273 SARS-CoV-2 vaccine. *Vaccine* 39(20):2791–2799.

Cobey, S., and S. E. Hensley. 2017. Immune history and influenza virus susceptibility. *Current Opinion in Virology* 22:105–111.

Coffman, R. L., A. Sher, and R. A. Seder. 2010. Vaccine adjuvants: Putting innate immunity to work. *Immunity* 33(4):492–503.

CONSISE (Consortium for the Standardization of Influenza Seroepidemiology). 2021. *About us*. https://consise.tghn.org/about (accessed October 19, 2021).

Corder, B. N., B. L. Bullard, G. A. Poland, and E. A. Weaver. 2020. A decade in review: A systematic review of universal influenza vaccines in clinical trials during the 2010 decade. *Viruses* 12(10):1186.

Cox, N. J., J. Hickling, R. Jones, G. F. Rimmelzwaan, L. C. Lambert, J. Boslego, L. Rudenko, L. Yeolekar, J. S. Robertson, J. Hombach, and J. R. Ortiz. 2015. Report on the second WHO integrated meeting on development and clinical trials of influenza vaccines that induce broadly protective and long-lasting immune responses. *Vaccine* 33(48):6503–6510.

DeMarcus, L., L. Shoubaki, and S. Federinko. 2019. Comparing influenza vaccine effectiveness between cell-derived and egg-derived vaccines, 2017–2018 influenza season. *Vaccine* 37(30):4015–4021.

Divino, V., G. Krishnarajah, S. I. Pelton, J. Mould-Quevedo, V. R. Anupindi, M. DeKoven, and M. J. Postma. 2020. A real-world study evaluating the relative vaccine effectiveness of a cell-based quadrivalent influenza vaccine compared to egg-based quadrivalent influenza vaccine in the US during the 2017–18 influenza season. *Vaccine* 38(40):6334–6343.

Dunkle, L. M., and R. Izikson. 2016. Recombinant hemagglutinin influenza vaccine provides broader spectrum protection. *Expert Review of Vaccines* 15(8):957–966.

Eisenstein, M. 2019. Towards a universal flu vaccine. *Nature* 573(7774):S50–S52.

Erbelding, E. J., D. J. Post, E. J. Stemmy, P. C. Roberts, A. D. Augustine, S. Ferguson, C. I. Paules, B. S. Graham, and A. S. Fauci. 2018. A universal influenza vaccine: The strategic plan for the National Institute of Allergy and Infectious Diseases. *Journal of Infectious Diseases* 218(3):347–354.

European Commission. 2021. *EU research and innovation supporting vaccine development for COVID-19*. https://ec.europa.eu/info/research-and-innovation/research-area/health-research-and-innovation/coronavirus-research-and-innovation/vaccines_en (accessed October 19, 2021).

FDA (U.S. Food and Drug Administration). 2015. *Drug development and review definitions*. https://www.fda.gov/drugs/investigational-new-drug-ind-application/drug-development-and-review-definitions (accessed October 19, 2021).

FDA. 2019. *First FDA-approved vaccine for the prevention of Ebola virus disease, marking a critical milestone in public health preparedness and response*. https://www.fda.gov/news-events/press-announcements/first-fda-approved-vaccine-prevention-ebola-virus-disease-marking-critical-milestone-public-health (accessed October 19, 2021).

FLUCOP Standardization and Development of Assays for Assessment of Influenza Vaccine Correlates of Protection. 2020. *Standardisation and development of assays for assessment of influenza vaccine correlates of protection*. https://flucop.eu (accessed October 19, 2021).

Fonville, J. M., S. H. Wilks, S. L. James, A. Fox, M. Ventresca, M. Aban, L. Xue, T. C. Jones, N. M. H. Le, Q. T. Pham, N. D. Tran, Y. Wong, A. Mosterin, L. C. Katzelnick, D. Labonte, T. T. Le, G. van der Net, E. Skepner, C. A. Russell, T. D. Kaplan, G. F. Rimmelzwaan, N. Masurel, J. C. de Jong, A. Palache, W. E. P. Beyer, Q. M. Le, T. H. Nguyen, H. F. L. Wertheim, A. C. Hurt, A. D. M. E. Osterhaus, I. G. Barr, R. A. M. Fouchier, P. W. Horby, and D. J. Smith. 2014. Antibody landscapes after influenza virus infection or vaccination. *Science* 346(6212):996–1000.

Francis, T. 1960. On the doctrine of original antigenic sin. *Proceedings of the American Philosophical Society* 104(6):572–578.

Friede, M., L. Palkonyay, C. Alfonso, Y. Pervikov, G. Torelli, D. Wood, and M. P. Kieny. 2011. WHO initiative to increase global and equitable access to influenza vaccine in the event of a pandemic: Supporting developing country production capacity through technology transfer. *Vaccine* 29:A2–A7.

GAO (U.S. Government Accountability Office). 2021. *Operation Warp Speed: Accelerated COVID-19 vaccine development status and efforts to address manufacturing challenges.* https://www.gao.gov/products/gao-21-319 (accessed October 19, 2021).

Gavi (The Vaccine Alliance). 2021. *The COVID-19 vaccine race—weekly update.* https://www.gavi.org/vaccineswork/covid-19-vaccine-race (accessed October 19, 2021).

Gomez Lorenzo, M. M., and M. J. Fenton. 2013. Immunobiology of influenza vaccines. *Chest* 143(2):502–510.

Gostic, K. M., M. Ambrose, M. Worobey, and J. O. Lloyd-Smith. 2016. Potent protection against H5N1 and H7N9 influenza via childhood hemagglutinin imprinting. *Science* 354(6313):722–726.

Gottlieb, T., and T. Ben-Yedidia. 2014. Epitope-based approaches to a universal influenza vaccine. *Journal of Autoimmunity* 54:15–20.

Gouglas, D., T. Thanh Le, K. Henderson, A. Kaloudis, T. Danielsen, N. C. Hammersland, J. M. Robinson, P. M. Heaton, and J.-A. Røttingen. 2018. Estimating the cost of vaccine development against epidemic infectious diseases: A cost minimisation study. *Lancet Global Health* 6(12):e1386–e1396.

Gouma, S., S. J. Zost, K. Parkhouse, A. Branche, D. J. Topham, S. Cobey, and S. E. Hensley. 2020. Comparison of human H3N2 antibody responses elicited by egg-based, cell-based, and recombinant protein-based influenza vaccines during the 2017-2018 season. *Clinical Infectious Diseases* 71(6):1447–1453.

GPMB (Global Preparedness Monitoring Board). 2019. *Pandemic preparedness financing status update.* https://www.gpmb.org/#tab=tab_1 (accessed October 19, 2021).

Graham, B. S. 2021. Lessons learned from COVID-19 for pandemic preparedness: Vaccine R&D for advancing pandemic and seasonal influenza preparedness, learning from the COVID-19 vaccine experience.

Hampson, A., I. Barr, N. Cox, R. O. Donis, S. Siddhivinayak, D. Jernigan, J. Katz, J. McCauley, F. Motta, T. Odagiri, J. S. Tam, A. Waddell, R. Webby, T. Ziegler, and W. Zhang. 2017. Improving the selection and development of influenza vaccine viruses—report of a WHO informal consultation on improving influenza vaccine virus selection, Hong Kong SAR, China, 18–20 November 2015. *Vaccine* 35(8):1104–1109.

Huang, K.-Y. A., S.-C. Chang, Y.-C. Huang, C.-H. Chiu, and T.-Y. Lin. 2017. Antibody responses to trivalent inactivated influenza vaccine in health care personnel previously vaccinated and vaccinated for the first time. *Scientific Reports* 7:40027.

IOM (Institute of Medicine). 2010. *The 2009 H1N1 influenza vaccination campaign: Summary of a workshop series.* Washington, DC: The National Academies Press.

IWG (International Working Group on Financing Preparedness). 2017. *From panic and neglect to investing in health security: Financing pandemic preparedness at a national level.* Washington, DC: World Bank Group.

Izurieta, H. S., Y. Chillarige, J. Kelman, Y. Wei, Y. Lu, W. Xu, M. Lu, D. Pratt, S. Chu, M. Wernecke, T. MaCurdy, and R. Forshee. 2018. Relative effectiveness of cell-cultured and egg-based influenza vaccines among elderly persons in the United States, 2017–2018. *Journal of Infectious Diseases* 220(8):1255–1264.

Jazayeri, S. D., and C. L. Poh. 2019. Development of universal influenza vaccines targeting conserved viral proteins. *Vaccines* 7(4):169.

Kelvin, A. A., and M. Zambon. 2019. Influenza imprinting in childhood and the influence on vaccine response later in life. *Euro Surveillance* 24(48):1900720.

Khoury, D. S., D. Cromer, A. Reynaldi, T. E. Schlub, A. K. Wheatley, J. A. Juno, K. Subbarao, S. J. Kent, J. A. Triccas, and M. P. Davenport. 2021. Neutralizing antibody levels are highly predictive of immune protection from symptomatic SARS-CoV-2 infection. *Nature Medicine* 27(7):1205–1211.

Klasse, P. J., D. F. Nixon, and J. P. Moore. 2021. Immunogenicity of clinically relevant SARS-CoV-2 vaccines in nonhuman primates and humans. *Science Advances* 7(12):eabe8065.

Klein, N. P., B. Fireman, K. Goddard, O. Zerbo, J. Asher, J. Zhou, J. King, and N. Lewis. 2020. Vaccine effectiveness of cell-culture relative to egg-based inactivated influenza vaccine during the 2017–18 influenza season. *PLOS ONE* 15(2):e0229279.

Knezevic, I., M. A. Liu, K. Peden, T. Zhou, and H. N. Kang. 2021. Development of mRNA vaccines: Scientific and regulatory issues. *Vaccines* 9(2):1–11.

Krammer, F. 2019. The human antibody response to influenza a virus infection and vaccination. *Nature Reviews Immunology* 19(6):383–397.

Krammer, F. 2020. SARS-CoV-2 vaccines in development. *Nature* 586(7830):516–527.

Krammer, F., and P. Palese. 2015. Advances in the development of influenza virus vaccines. *Nature Reviews Drug Discovery* 14(3):167–182.

Krishnarajah, G., V. Divino, M. J. Postma, S. I. Pelton, V. R. Anupindi, M. DeKoven, and J. Mould-Quevedo. 2021. Clinical and economic outcomes associated with cell-based quadrivalent influenza vaccine vs. standard-dose egg-based quadrivalent influenza vaccines during the 2018–19 influenza season in the United States. *Vaccines* 9(2):80.

Lederer, K., D. Castaño, D. Gómez Atria, T. H. Oguin 3rd, S. Wang, T. B. Manzoni, H. Muramatsu, M. J. Hogan, F. Amanat, P. Cherubin, K. A. Lundgreen, Y. K. Tam, S. H. Y. Fan, L. C. Eisenlohr, I. Maillard, D. Weissman, P. Bates, F. Krammer, G. D. Sempowski, N. Pardi, and M. Locci. 2020. SARS-CoV-2 mRNA vaccines foster potent antigen-specific germinal center responses associated with neutralizing antibody generation. *Immunity* 53(6):1281–1295.

Leung, V. K. Y., A. Fox, L. A. Carolan, M. Aban, K. L. Laurie, J. Druce, Y.-M. Deng, M. A. Slavin, C. Marshall, and S. G. Sullivan. 2021. Impact of prior vaccination on antibody response and influenza-like illness among Australian healthcare workers after influenza vaccination in 2016. *Vaccine* 39(24):3270–3278.

Lim, W. W., N. H. L. Leung, S. G. Sullivan, E. J. Tchetgen, and B. J. Cowling. 2020. Distinguishing causation from correlation in the use of correlates of protection to evaluate and develop influenza vaccines. *American Journal of Epidemiology* 189(3):185–192.

Logunov, D. Y., I. V. Dolzhikova, D. V. Shcheblyakov, A. I. Tukhvatulin, O. V. Zubkova, A. S. Dzharullaeva, A. V. Kovyrshina, N. L. Lubenets, D. M. Grousova, A. S. Erokhova, A. G. Botikov, F. M. Izhaeva, O. Popova, T. A. Ozharovskaya, I. B. Esmagambetov, I. A. Favorskaya, D. I. Zrelkin, D. V. Voronina, D. N. Shcherbinin, A. S. Semikhin, Y. V. Simakova, E. A. Tokarskaya, D. A. Egorova, M. M. Shmarov, N. A. Nikitenko, V. A. Gushchin, E. A. Smolyarchuk, S. K. Zyryanov, S. V. Borisevich, B. S. Naroditsky, and A. L. Gintsburg. 2021. Safety and efficacy of an RAD26 and RAD5 vector-based heterologous prime-boost COVID-19 vaccine: An interim analysis of a randomised controlled phase 3 trial in Russia. *Lancet* 397(10275):671–681.

Milián, E., and A. A. Kamen. 2015. Current and emerging cell culture manufacturing technologies for influenza vaccines. *BioMedical Research International* 2015.

Mishra, M. 2021. *World to spend $157 billion on COVID-19 vaccines through 2025 report.* https://www.reuters.com/business/healthcare-pharmaceuticals/world-spend-157-billion-covid-19-vaccines-through-2025-report-2021-04-29 (accessed October 19, 2021).

Mohn, K. G. I., I. Smith, H. Sjursen, and R. J. Cox. 2018. Immune responses after live attenuated influenza vaccination. *Human Vaccines & Immunotherapeutics* 14(3):571–578.

Morimoto, N., and K. Takeishi. 2018. Change in the efficacy of influenza vaccination after repeated inoculation under antigenic mismatch: A systematic review and meta-analysis. *Vaccine* 36(7):949–957.

Mosterín Höpping, A., J. McElhaney, J. M. Fonville, D. C. Powers, W. E. P. Beyer, and D. J. Smith. 2016. The confounded effects of age and exposure history in response to influenza vaccination. *Vaccine* 34(4):540–546.

Nachbagauer, R., and F. Krammer. 2017. Universal influenza virus vaccines and therapeutic antibodies. *Clinical Microbiology and Infection* 23(4):222–228.

NAM (National Academy of Medicine). 2016. *The neglected dimension of global security: A framework to counter infectious disease crises*. Washington, DC: The National Academies Press. Pp. 17–22.

NCIRS (National Centre for Immunisation Research and Surveillance). 2020. *Phases of clinical trials* https://www.ncirs.org.au/phases-clinical-trials (accessed October 19, 2021).

Newland, M., D. Durham, J. Asher, J. J. Treanor, J. Seals, R. O. Donis, and R. A. Johnson. 2021. Improving pandemic preparedness through better, faster influenza vaccines. *Expert Review of Vaccines*.

Nguyen-Contant, P., M. Y. Sangster, and D. J. Topham. 2021. Squalene-based influenza vaccine adjuvants and their impact on the hemagglutinin-specific B cell response. *Pathogens* 10(3):355.

NIAID (National Institute of Allergy and Infectious Diseases). 2021. *NIAID strategic plan for a universal influenza vaccine*. https://www.niaidcivics.org/news/2019/10/niaid-strategic-plan-for-a-universal-influenza-vaccine (accessed October 19, 2021).

NIH (National Institutes of Health). 2021. https://clinicaltrials.gov/ct2/results/map?term=universal+influenza+vaccine&map= (accessed October 19, 2021).

Novavax. 2021. *Novavax COVID-19 vaccine demonstrates 90% overall efficacy and 100% protection against moderate and severe disease in prevent-19 phase 3 trial*. Gaithersburg, MD: Novavax, Inc.

Oliver, S. E., J. W. Gargano, H. Scobie, M. Wallace, S. C. Hadler, J. Leung, A. E. Blain, N. McClung, D. Campos-Outcalt, R. L. Morgan, S. Mbaeyi, J. MacNeil, J. R. Romero, H. K. Talbot, G. M. Lee, B. P. Bell, and K. Dooling. 2021. The advisory committee on immunization practices' interim recommendation for use of Janssen COVID-19 vaccine—United States, February 2021. *Morbidity and Mortality Weekly Report* 70(9):329–332.

PATH. 2020. *Vaccine cold chain Q&A*. https://www.path.org/articles/vaccine-cold-chain-q (accessed October 19, 2021).

Paules, C. I., and A. S. Fauci. 2019. Influenza vaccines: Good, but we can do better. *Journal of Infectious Diseases* 219(Suppl 1):S1–S4.

Paules, C. I., S. G. Sullivan, K. Subbarao, and A. S. Fauci. 2017. Chasing seasonal influenza—the need for a universal influenza vaccine. *New England Journal of Medicine* 378(1):7–9.

Peshimam, G. N., and U. Farooq. 2021. CanSinoBio's COVID-19 vaccine 65.7% effective in global trials, Pakistan official says. *Reuters*. https://www.reuters.com/article/us-health-coronavirus-vaccine-pakistan/cansinobios-covid-19-vaccine-65-7-effective-in-global-trials-pakistan-official-says-idUSKBN2A81N0 (accessed October 19, 2021).

Plotkin, S., J. M. Robinson, G. Cunningham, R. Iqbal, and S. Larsen. 2017. The complexity and cost of vaccine manufacturing - An overview. *Vaccine* 35(33):4064–4071.

Pokharel, K. 2021. *India's Bharat Biotech says vaccine is effective against delta variant*. https://www.wsj.com/articles/indias-bharat-biotech-says-vaccine-is-effective-against-delta-variant-11625325879 (accessed October 19, 2021).

Polack, F. P., S. J. Thomas, N. Kitchin, J. Absalon, A. Gurtman, S. Lockhart, J. L. Prez, G. Pérez Marc, E. D. Moreira, C. Zerbini, R. Bailey, K. A. Swanson, S. Roychoudhury, K. Koury, P. Li, W. V. Kalina, D. Cooper, R. W. Frenck, L. L. Hammitt, Ö. Türeci, H. Nell, A. Schaefer, S. Ünal, D. B. Tresnan, S. Mather, P. R. Dormitzer, U. Şahin, K. U. Jansen, and W. C. Gruber. 2020. Safety and efficacy of the BNT162b2 mRNA COVID-19 vaccine. *New England Journal of Medicine* 383(27):2603–2615.

Pollet, J., W.-H. Chen, and U. Strych. 2021. Recombinant protein vaccines, a proven approach against coronavirus pandemics. *Advanced Drug Delivery Reviews* 170:71–82.

Rajaram, S., C. Boikos, D. K. Gelone, and A. Gandhi. 2020a. Influenza vaccines: The potential benefits of cell-culture isolation and manufacturing. *Therapeutic Advances in Vaccines and Immunotherapy* 8:2515135520908121.

Rajaram, S., R. Wojcik, C. Moore, R. Ortiz de Lejarazu, S. de Lusignan, E. Montomoli, A. Rossi, A. Pérez-Rubio, A. Trilla, V. Baldo, R. Jandhyala, and G. Kassianos. 2020b. The impact of candidate influenza virus and egg-based manufacture on vaccine effectiveness: Literature review and expert consensus. *Vaccine* 38(38):6047–6056.

Rappuoli, R., and P. R. Dormitzer. 2012. Influenza: Options to improve pandemic preparation. *Science* 336(6088):1531–1533.

Reber, A. J., T. Chirkova, J. H. Kim, W. Cao, R. Biber, D. K. Shay, and S. Sambhara. 2012. Immunosenescence and challenges of vaccination against influenza in the aging population. *Aging and Disease* 3(1):68–90.

Rockman, S., K. L. Laurie, S. Parkes, A. Wheatley, and I. G. Barr. 2020. New technologies for influenza vaccines. *Microorganisms* 8(11):1745.

Rosa, S. S., D. M. F. Prazeres, A. M. Azevedo, and M. P. C. Marques. 2021. mRNA vaccines manufacturing: Challenges and bottlenecks. *Vaccine* 39(16):2190–2200.

Ruiz-Aragón, J., R. Gani, S. Márquez, and P. Alvarez. 2020. Estimated cost-effectiveness and burden of disease associated with quadrivalent cell-based and egg-based influenza vaccines in spain. *Human Vaccines & Immunotherapeutics* 16(9):2238-2244.

Saif, L. J. 2020. Vaccines for COVID-19: Perspectives, prospects, and challenges based on candidate SARS, MERS, and animal coronavirus vaccines. *European Medical Journal*. March 24.

Saito, N., K. Komori, M. Suzuki, K. Morimoto, T. Kishikawa, T. Yasaka, and K. Ariyoshi. 2017. Negative impact of prior influenza vaccination on current influenza vaccination among people infected and not infected in prior season: A test-negative case-control study in japan. *Vaccine* 35(4):687–693.

Sanofi. 2021. Sanofi and GSK initiate global phase 3 clinical efficacy study of COVID-19 vaccine candidate. May 27, 2021. https://www.sanofi.com/en/media-room/press-releases/2021/2021-05-27-07-30-00-2236989#:~:text=Home-,Sanofi%20and%20GSK%20initiate%20global%20Phase%203%20clinical,of%20COVID%2D19%20vaccine%20candidate&text=PARIS%20and%20LONDON%20%E2%80%93%20May%2027,protein%20COVID%2D19%20vaccine%20candidate (accessed October 19, 2021).

Saville, M. 2021. Presentation. Updated figure provided by Coalition for Epidemic Preparedness.

Scripps Research Institute. 2017. *How flu shot manufacturing forces influenza to mutate: Egg-based production causes virus to target bird cells, making vaccine less effective*. https://www.sciencedaily.com/releases/2017/10/171030134625.htm (accessed October 19, 2021).

Slaoui, M., and M. Hepburn. 2020. Developing safe and effective COVID vaccines—Operation Warp Speed's strategy and approach. *New England Journal of Medicine* 383(18):1701–1703.

Sparrow, E., J. G. Wood, C. Chadwick, A. T. Newall, S. Torvaldsen, A. Moen, and G. Torelli. 2021. Global production capacity of seasonal and pandemic influenza vaccines in 2019. *Vaccine* 39(3):512–520.

Stowe, J., N. Andrews, C. Gower, E. Gallagher, L. Utsi, R. Simmons, S. Thelwall, E. Tessier, N. Groves, G. Dabrera, R. Myers, C. Campbell, G. Amirthalingham, M. Edmuds, M. Zambon, K. Brown, S. Hopkins, M. Chand, M. Ramsay, and J. Lopez Bernal. 2021. Effectiveness of COVID-19 vaccines against hospital admission with the delta (b.1.617.2) variant. *Public Health England*.

Subbarao, K. 2021. The success of SARS-CoV-2 vaccines and challenges ahead. *Cell Host Microbe* 29(7):1111–1123.

Sullivan, S. G., S. Feng, and B. J. Cowling. 2014. Potential of the test-negative design for measuring influenza vaccine effectiveness: A systematic review. *Expert Review of Vaccines* 13(12):1571–1591.

Thompson, M. G., A. Naleway, A. M. Fry, S. Ball, S. M. Spencer, S. Reynolds, S. Bozeman, M. Levine, J. M. Katz, and M. Gaglani. 2016. Effects of repeated annual inactivated influenza vaccination among healthcare personnel on serum hemagglutinin inhibition antibody response to A/Perth/16/2009 (H3N2)-like virus during 2010–11. *Vaccine* 34(7):981–988.

Ulmer, J. B., U. Valley, and R. Rappuoli. 2006. Vaccine manufacturing: Challenges and solutions. *Nature Biotechnology* 24(11):1377–1383.

Vasireddy, D., P. Atluri, S. V. Malayala, R. Vanaparthy, and G. Mohan. 2021. Review of COVID-19 vaccines approved in the United States of America for emergency use. *Journal of Clinical Medicine Research* 13(4):204–213.

Voysey, M., S. A. C. Clemens, S. A. Madhi, L. Y. Weckx, P. M. Folegatti, P. K. Aley, B. Angus, V. L. Baillie, S. L. Barnabas, Q. E. Bhorat, S. Bibi, C. Briner, P. Cicconi, A. M. Collins, R. Colin-Jones, C. L. Cutland, T. C. Darton, K. Dheda, C. J. A. Duncan, et al. 2021. Safety and efficacy of the ChAdOx1 nCoV-19 vaccine (AZD1222) against SARS-CoV-2: An interim analysis of four randomised controlled trials in Brazil, South Africa, and the UK. *Lancet* 397(10269):99–111.

Wang, W., E. Alvarado-Facundo, R. Vassell, L. Collins, R. E. Colombo, A. Ganesan, C. Geaney, D. Hrncir, T. Lalani, A. E. Markelz, R. C. Maves, B. McClenathan, K. Mende, S. A. Richard, C. Schofield, S. Seshadri, C. Spooner, G. C. Utz, T. E. Warkentien, M. Levine, C. L. Coles, T. H. Burgess, M. Eichelberger, and C. D. Weiss. 2020. Comparison of A(H3N2) neutralizing antibody responses elicited by 2018–2019 season quadrivalent influenza vaccines derived from eggs, cells, and recombinant hemagglutinin. *Clinical Infectious Diseases*. September 8.

Wei, C.-J., M. C. Crank, J. Shiver, B. S. Graham, J. R. Mascola, and G. J. Nabel. 2020. Next-generation influenza vaccines: Opportunities and challenges. *Nature Reviews Drug Discovery* 19(4):239–252.

Weir, J. P., and M. F. Gruber. 2016. An overview of the regulation of influenza vaccines in the United States. *Influenza and Other Respiratory Viruses* 10(5):354–360.

WHO (World Health Organization). 2021a. *WHO coronavirus (COVID-19) dashboard.* https://covid19.who.int (accessed October 19, 2021).

WHO. 2021b. *WHO validates Sinovac COVID-19 vaccine for emergency use and issues interim policy recommendations.* https://www.who.int/news/item/01-06-2021-who-validates-sinovac-covid-19-vaccine-for-emergency-use-and-issues-interim-policy-recommendations (accessed October 19, 2021).

Wong, S.-S., and R. J. Webby. 2013. Traditional and new influenza vaccines. *Clinical Microbiology Reviews* 26(3):476–492.

Wright, P. F. 2008. Vaccine preparedness—are we ready for the next influenza pandemic? *New England Journal of Medicine* 358(24):2540–2543.

Wu, K., A. P. Werner, J. I. Moliva, M. Koch, A. Choi, G. B. E. Stewart-Jones, H. Bennett, S. Boyoglu-Barnum, W. Shi, B. S. Graham, A. Carfi, K. S. Corbett, R. A. Seder, and D. K. Edwards. 2021. mRNA-1273 vaccine induces neutralizing antibodies against spike mutants from global SARS-CoV-2 variants. *bioRxiv*. January 25.

Zeigler, D. F., E. Gage, and C. H. Clegg. 2021. Epitope-targeting platform for broadly protective influenza vaccines. *PLOS ONE* 16(5):e0252170.

Zimmer, C., and K. Thomas. 2020. Was the Pfizer vaccine part of the government's Operation Warp Speed? *The New York Times*. November 10.

Zimmer, C., J. Corum, and S.-L. Wee. 2021. *Coronavirus vaccine tracker*. https://www.nytimes.com/interactive/2020/science/coronavirus-vaccine-tracker.html (accessed October 19, 2021).

Zost, S. J., K. Parkhouse, M. E. Gumina, K. Kim, S. Diaz Perez, P. C. Wilson, J. J. Treanor, A. J. Sant, S. Cobey, and S. E. Hensley. 2017. Contemporary H3N2 influenza viruses have a glycosylation site that alters binding of antibodies elicited by egg-adapted vaccine strains. *Proceedings of the National Academy of Sciences* 114(47):12578–12583.

3

Clinical Science

This chapter addresses the second of the four dimensions of vaccine research, development, and manufacturing examined by the committee. It begins by describing the role of clinical science in the development of COVID-19 vaccines. The chapter then considers how lessons learned from the development of COVID-19 vaccines (shown in Box 3-1) can be applied to both seasonal and pandemic influenza vaccines in the dimension of clinical science. The final section presents recommendations drawn from these findings.

BOX 3-1
Clinical Science: Lessons Learned from the COVID-19 Pandemic

- Coordination between vaccine manufacturers and regulatory authorities ensured seamless transition between immunogenicity and efficacy trials and the clinical testing phase, significantly speeding up the process.
- While many vaccine trials aimed to include participants of all ages, races, ethnicities, minorities, and the elderly, some populations (e.g., children, pregnant people) were not included early on.
- At-risk populations, such as the immunocompromised and the elderly, must be prioritized during vaccine distribution.
- Pharmacovigilance surveillance, both during clinical trials and postauthorization, is critical for detecting rare but severe vaccine safety signals.
- Funding from public–private partnerships assisted manufacturers in overcoming cost barriers to developing novel vaccines for COVID-19, allowing novel platforms such as mRNA to be explored.

CLINICAL SCIENCE AND THE DEVELOPMENT OF COVID-19 VACCINES

Lessons can be learned from the experience with developing COVID-19 vaccines in several aspects of clinical science: preclinical and clinical trial design, diversity in clinical trials, evaluation of vaccine effectiveness (VE), and postauthorization safety surveillance.

Preclinical and Clinical Trial Design

During a pandemic, when speed is of the essence, vaccine development through clinical testing in the traditional, sequential order is time consuming. To allow the unprecedented rapid vaccine development for COVID-19, vaccine manufacturers conducted immunogenicity and efficacy trials in parallel, instead of the traditional sequential path of studies (Excler et al., 2021). A data and safety monitoring board (DSMB) was formed to evaluate government-funded trials, coordinate oversight, and share learning pertaining to safety across trials. Additionally, manufacturers liaised with regulatory bodies to clearly define expectations and expedite the process to authorization. Regulatory systems that laid out clear guidelines and worked closely together with industry facilitated these overlapping preclinical and clinical phase studies, while maintaining regulatory standards (see Chapter 5).

The U.S. Food and Drug Administration (FDA) approved Emergency Use Authorization for those vaccines that showed an efficacy of at least 50 percent in placebo-controlled phase III trials and were considered safe (FDA, 2021a). The European Medicines Agency (EMA) had a conditional marketing authorization in place to enable authorization as soon as sufficient data were available regarding efficacy and safety, while requiring monthly safety reports from manufacturers (EMA, 2021a,b). Additionally, regulators allowed for a rolling review of data during the developmental stages of the vaccines to further accelerate the process.

Vaccines should be made available to the most at-risk populations first. Therefore, careful attention should be given to the design and inclusion criteria in trials to allow the vaccine to be available to the most at-risk populations first. In the COVID-19 pandemic, populations at highest risk of disease and death were largely composed of older adults, with 80 percent of deaths occurring in adults over 65 years of age (CDC, 2021a). As a result, vaccine trials—and ultimately vaccine distribution—prioritized these individuals, including first responders, older adults, those with chronic conditions, and marginalized populations that were disproportionately affected by the pandemic (Dooling et al., 2021; Soiza et al., 2021). Especially as it relates to the latter, there was unprecedented advocacy for the engagement of diverse populations, although, as discussed below, most clinical trials ultimately fell short in this regard, and many minority populations were underrepresented (Flores et al., 2021). The goal was three-fold: to learn whether the vaccine candidates were safe, to assess whether they were effective at preventing disease, and to educate these communities about the anticipated benefits of vaccination. While these efforts were generally successful, segments of these communities continue to experience vaccine hesitancy despite the availability of safe and effective vaccines against COVID-19 (Razai et al., 2021).

Diversity in Clinical Trials

Historically, diversity among participants in clinical trials examining vaccine safety and efficacy has not reflected the diversity of the population. In the United States, in a study comparing clinical trial data, it was found that out of 230 trials, only 58.3 percent reported on race and 34.2 percent on ethnicity (Flores et al., 2021). White people were overrepresented in these studies, while Black people were underrepresented. Additionally, the distribution of age groups also does not match their distribution in the population, with those over 65 making up just 12.1 percent of study populations (Flores et al., 2021). Yet, to obtain accurate estimates of efficacy, diversity in enrollment for clinical trials for vaccines is required, including all populations at risk, such as people of all ages and pregnant people.

COVID-19 has disproportionally affected various racial and ethnic groups and is more severe in older adults and those with preexisting conditions (Garg et al., 2020; Webb Hooper et al., 2020). While minorities and the elderly were underrepresented in clinical trials, people who were known to be pregnant were excluded altogether from the phase III efficacy clinical trials for the COVID-19 vaccines (Subbaraman, 2021; Van Spall, 2021). Therefore, limited data were available for recommendations at the time of Emergency Use Authorization. However, given that COVID-19 poses risks for pregnancy outcomes, in most countries, people who were pregnant were offered the vaccine. Monitoring studies are ongoing, and early results suggest the vaccines are safe and effective in this group. Recent data show that in a cohort of 103 women receiving mRNA vaccination, 30 of whom were pregnant and 16 lactating, immunogenicity was similar in all women, and vaccine-induced antibodies were found in their cord blood and breast milk (Collier et al., 2021). Another study among 84 women who received the vaccine during pregnancy showed the vaccine was not associated with placental histopathologic lesions (Shanes et al., 2021).

Children younger than 16 years were also not included in the initial phase III efficacy trials for these vaccines. On the basis of these trial data, the Moderna and Johnson & Johnson vaccines were authorized for ages 18 and older, while the Pfizer-BioNTech vaccine was approved for those 16 and older in most countries (AJMC Staff, 2021a,b). Clinical trials including adolescents followed the successful phase III studies, and Pfizer-BioNTech was authorized for use in children aged 12–15 years in the United States in May 2021 (AJMC Staff, 2021b). Trials for AstraZeneca in children have been halted pending a safety review after rare cases of blood clots in the brain were reported in adult trials (Cunningham and Iati, 2021).

Postauthorization Vaccine Safety Surveillance

A critical component of global vaccination efforts is the ability to monitor vaccine safety in real time. Investment in vaccine safety surveillance systems is crucial to achieve three goals:

1. Support streamlined vaccine development;
2. Promote confidence in vaccines; and
3. Ensure trust in decision making about vaccine use by enabling dynamic benefit–risk assessments.

Clinical trials are typically designed to evaluate efficacy or immunogenicity and are usually sufficient in size to detect common adverse events, such as local or systemic reactogenicity. However, clinical trials are often not powered to detect rare, significant adverse events. A notable exception is the rotavirus vaccine, where pre-licensure trials for subsequent rotavirus vaccines were a priori designed to demonstrate that the risk of intussusception was similar in vaccine versus placebo recipients following observations of intussusception with rotavirus vaccine (Heyse et al., 2008).

Passive surveillance systems, such as the Vaccine Adverse Event Reporting System (VAERS) used in the United States, enable reporting of potential adverse events to a public health authority and can be efficient and timely for detecting rare adverse events (Cashman et al., 2017; Chandler, 2020; Gee et al., 2021; Zanardi et al., 2001). Active monitoring systems, such as the Vaccine Safety Datalink (VSD), are coordinated by the U.S. Centers for Disease Control and Prevention (CDC) and other health systems that assess population-based data with appropriate comparison groups to estimate burden and risk in different populations using electronic medical records and health care encounter data (Lee et al., 2020). Certain population-based surveillance systems include the use of electronic medical records, which is critical for signal validation (FDA, 2021b; Nsubuga et al., 2006; Remmel, 2021). However, these are less commonly available for use as a component of vaccine safety surveillance programs in many countries. Clinical consultation services have also been extremely useful to complement existing safety surveillance systems in the United States and to better support causality assessment of safety signals (Buehler et al., 2004). The vaccine safety review process can also include informal sources, such as social media, watchlists, global and regional databases; formal sources, such as global databases of case safety reports and regional databases; and routine meetings with various regulators—such as the International Coalition of Medicines Regulatory Authorities (ICRMA), FDA, EMA, and low- and middle-income countries (LMICs) having weekly huddles with all six World Health Organization (WHO) regional offices (Helfand and Pal, 2021).

Clinical trials for COVID-19 vaccines were unusual in size, speed, and diverse enrollment practices. To rapidly evaluate the efficacy of newer platforms used for vaccine development, trials contained more than 30,000 participants in the pivotal phase III clinical trials in adult populations (Brothers, 2020; May, 2020; Pfizer, 2020). Given the large size of these initial trials, regulatory agencies in the United States prespecified that a median of 2 months of safety follow-up was sufficient to apply for Emergency Use Authorization, balancing the need for timely availability of vaccines with the ability to detect common vaccine safety events (FDA, 2021a). Subsequent trials, however, are likely to rely on immunobridging rather than efficacy data, deducing efficacy in different populations. This may limit risk–benefit analysis and the availability of safety data in subpopulations such as young children.

As humans are naïve to SARS-CoV-2, potential safety signals for the vaccines were initially unknown. However, efforts have been made to identify and prepare for potential side effects. The Safety Platform for Emergency vACcines (SPEAC) project was formed by the Coalition for Epidemic Preparedness Innovations (CEPI) and the Brighton Collaboration in an attempt to create a list of potential adverse events of special interest following COVID-19 vaccination and how to respond appropriately to such adverse events should they occur (Black et al., 2021).

While clinical trials result in a reasonable degree of certainty about the frequency of common adverse events in the overall population such as local and systemic reactogenicity, postauthorization or postapproval safety surveillance systems can affirm that the risk is similar across diverse, real-world populations, meaning by age (teens, elderly), gender, race/ethnicity, presence of comorbidities, and pregnancy. During the COVID-19 pandemic, a novel safety surveillance system called v-safe was implemented using smartphone technology, allowing vaccine recipients to directly report potential adverse events to public health agencies

(CDC, 2021b; Gee et al., 2021). Text messaging reminders and links to web surveys enabled vaccine recipients in the United States to record their symptoms following vaccination and report any health impact events. Furthermore, a pregnancy v-safe registry was launched in the United States when it was noted that more pregnant individuals received COVID-19 vaccines early in the pandemic than anticipated (more than 150,000 as of August 2021), in the paucity of clinical trial data (CDC, 2021c). Pregnant individuals had comparable reactogenicity to non-pregnant individuals (Shimabukuro et al., 2021). More than 5,000 of these women have volunteered to provide additional data on their pregnancy and neonatal outcomes (CDC, 2021c). These data could potentially support expanded use of vaccines in different countries where variation in policies or recommendations owing to concerns about safety issues may affect access to vaccines (COMIT, 2021).

Similar survey-based approaches to monitoring postauthorization or postapproval vaccine safety can provide data complementary to those obtained from clinical trials. For example, during COVID-19 vaccine trials, self-reported surveys were used to measure safety and reactogenicity. The study showed that more severe adverse events were more likely in participants who had previously been infected with SARS-CoV-2 (Mathioudakis et al., 2021). Similar results have been demonstrated in influenza vaccine studies, such as a short-term reactogenicity study after receiving a two-dose H5N1 vaccine (Standaert et al., 2019), and a study that sent participants a daily SMS link to collect reactogenicity data after vaccination (Stuurman et al., 2017).

In contrast to local and systemic reactogenicity, rare adverse events are difficult to detect in clinical trials. Instead, it is necessary to rely almost entirely on postauthorization or postapproval safety surveillance systems to capture rare adverse events. The importance of these systems during a pandemic cannot be overemphasized given our experience with observations of Guillain-Barré syndrome during the 1976 swine flu and 2009 H1N1 pandemics (Salmon et al., 2011; Sencer and Millar, 2006). During the vaccine rollout for COVID-19, some very rare adverse events have been detected, including anaphylaxis and myocarditis following receipt of the mRNA vaccines (Blumenthal et al., 2021; Kim et al., 2021) and thrombosis with thrombocytopenia syndrome (TTS) following receipt of the adenoviral vector-based vaccines (Meredith, 2021). These events have mainly been detected in countries with well-developed surveillance mechanisms and ongoing real-time monitoring and coordination between regulatory bodies within and across countries to ensure the rapid detection and management of these rare events. However, these surveillance systems may not accurately measure the experience of diverse populations receiving vaccines.

CLINICAL SCIENCE: APPLYING LESSONS FROM THE DEVELOPMENT OF COVID-19 VACCINES TO VACCINES FOR INFLUENZA

Diversity in Clinical Trials

When faced with an influenza pandemic, it is likely that the same diverse populations sought for COVID-19 vaccine trials, as well as the immunocompromised, children, and pregnant individuals, would benefit from vaccination at the earliest opportunity (Rasmussen et al., 2008; Ruf and Knuf, 2014). Therefore, diversity in clinical trials for influenza vaccines is critical as was the case with COVID-19 vaccines. Given the relatively low vaccination rates against seasonal influenza in pregnant individuals and children, it is reasonable to assume that there may be similar challenges in pandemic conditions (CDC, 2016, 2020).

Until recently, influenza vaccines have been implemented using a one-size-fits-all approach. However, the response to vaccines can vary with age. For instance, older individuals often have reduced responses to vaccines and might benefit from a higher vaccine dose or an adjuvanted vaccine to improve effectiveness in this population (Derhovanessian and Pawelec, 2012). Children who are naïve to influenza need to be primed suitably, which might be achieved with a live-attenuated vaccine that exposes them to all components of the influenza virus (Sridhar et al., 2015). Therefore, clinical vaccine platform development needs to consider the different needs of subsets of the population and incorporate them into the design of subsequent efficacy trials.

Clinical Trials for Influenza in Low- and Middle-Income Countries

The issue of clinical trials in LMICs is an important concern in the development of seasonal and pandemic influenza vaccines. The conduct of clinical trials and participation may be more problematic in LMICs where there are limited seasonal influenza programs due to lack of funds and a lack of urgency, as other health-related issues may take priority (Kraigsley et al., 2021; Ortiz and Neuzil, 2019; Williams et al., 2021). There may be limited surveillance data to support the need for vaccination in these areas. Moreover, even after the need is established, vaccine hesitancy may persist in the absence of local efficacy and safety data; limited capacity to distribute vaccines can also hamper efforts to increase vaccine coverage (Ortiz and Neuzil, 2019).

Conclusion 3-1: In LMICs that have performed disease burden studies, vaccination rates have improved (Bresee et al., 2018). Moreover, local surveillance data may convince local governments to invest in access to a seasonal vaccine and aid in increasing acceptability by the population. These strategies to increase seasonal influenza vaccine uptake would create a foundation for later introduction of pandemic influenza vaccines when they are needed.

Multiple factors may challenge the conduct of clinical trials in LMICs. First, clinical trial protocols need to be reviewed locally, which requires local expert committees. In outbreak situations, there is a risk that such committees may have limited capacity and can become overwhelmed. A lack of resources and expertise may limit the conduct of a prompt and complete review to assess the risks of the research and balance it with the risk of disease. Second, obtaining informed consent can be challenging in regions with low literacy levels, as there might be limited comprehension of the research principles, requiring witnesses and a more extensive consent process to explain the multitude of factors involved in the research (Minnies et al., 2008). Additionally, in many cultures, women are not the primary decision makers and might have lower levels of literacy (NBAC, 2001). Therefore, it can be challenging to include women or their children in trials. Third, specimen banking is often needed for clinical trials, which might not be possible in LMIC regions (Alemayehu et al., 2018). Additionally, certain levels of expertise might be needed to conduct assays on such samples, which might not be available in LMICs. Shipping specimen abroad to high-income countries for storage and analyses may also result in ownership issues.

Conclusion 3-2: The highest priority regions for vaccines are those where they are needed the most, the population at risk is willing to accept them, and local authorities can see their benefit. To achieve this goal, it is necessary to conduct clinical trials that include particularly at-risk populations. Local research centers in LMICs can conduct these trials, but the present model of providing temporary funding for specific projects for a limited amount of time makes it difficult to maintain them. As a result, it is challenging to quickly ramp up research efforts when there is a pandemic. During the COVID-19 pandemic, setting up and running trials of candidate vaccines has been slower in some areas of the world and is affecting uptake of these vaccines (COVID Clinical Research Coalition, 2020; Hall et al., 2021).

Monitoring Vaccine Effectiveness

For existing vaccine platforms, licensure of seasonal or pandemic influenza vaccines can be obtained either through a traditional approval pathway or by the accelerated approval mechanism (Weir and Gruber, 2016).

Typically, new vaccine platforms would use the traditional pathway and provide information on efficacy against influenza illness in clinical trials; however efficacy trials can be challenging to implement in a pandemic scenario where timeliness matters. Under the accelerated pathway, immunogenicity endpoints may be used for licensure as a mechanism for streamlining the vaccine approval process, with a requirement for postmarketing First Occurrence VE studies (Weir and Gruber, 2016).

While the appropriate pathway for regulatory approval for a pandemic influenza vaccine cannot be predicted, postmarket vaccine effectiveness evaluations are clearly needed for pandemic planning. Furthermore, ensuring that diverse populations are captured by these data systems is essential for a thorough assessment of the effectiveness of different vaccine platforms, adjuvants, doses, and schedules for different subpopulations, as well as effectiveness among emerging variants in the case of COVID-19.

VE studies are necessary for validating clinical trial data that may rely on immunogenicity or efficacy in well-defined populations. Real-world effectiveness may differ from prelicensure expectations, which in turn may affect benefit–risk balance and decision making about use of a vaccine in different populations (Hodgson et al., 2021). Efficiency in surveillance efforts is also essential for feasibility and sustainability. Previous work has provided some good models for VE studies, which can be applied to improving vaccines that target seasonal and pandemic influenza. The test-negative study design has been found to be an accurate way to monitor VE (Sullivan et al., 2014). This study design is a variant of the case-control study and is relatively easy to conduct, allowing its widespread use. It corrects for bias in health care–seeking behavior, as it studies those seeking health care for influenza-like symptoms (Jackson et al., 2006; Sullivan et al., 2014). Those who test positive for influenza infection are considered cases, and those who test negative serve as the controls. The vaccination status between the two groups is compared to determine the VE. This VE is estimated from the adjusted odds ratio and adjusts for potential confounders (Sullivan et al., 2014). The test-negative study design can be used to establish accurate VE for influenza vaccines.

Like clinical trials, VE studies need to include a representative mix of varying demographics (age, comorbidities, race/ethnicity); necessary as well is the standardization of age bands to provide accurate age estimates that can be applied to the population as a whole. Note that age affects VE for influenza and may bias VE assessment if not explicitly considered (Feng et al., 2021). Therefore, it may be preferable and more accurate to establish an age-weighted average VE to determine overall VE, instead of using the average without taking age into account.

Once a vaccine is licensed for use, yearly updates for strain changes can be submitted as a supplement to an existing license, without postmarket requirements for inactivated and recombinant protein vaccines (Wei et al., 2020). For example, 2009 monovalent H1N1 influenza vaccines were approved as a supplement to seasonal influenza vaccine licenses. Clinical trials to assess efficacy were not required prior to approval, shortening the time to an available H1N1 vaccine (Weir and Gruber, 2016). A similar approach to ensure timely access could be used for pandemic vaccines that are already licensed for use, with a supplement submitted for a strain change. In the absence of clinical efficacy data for a pandemic vaccine before authorization or approval, however, it becomes crucial to monitor vaccine effectiveness to support vaccine confidence and dynamic assessments of the benefit–risk balance.

The COVID-19 vaccine development story is remarkable. Novel platforms were evaluated for efficacy and safety in large-scale clinical trials prior to submission for Emergency Use Authorization, and the scope and speed of these clinical trials and the rapid regulatory response were unprecedented. In tandem with vaccine research, potential treatments for COVID-19 are also being explored. The WHO-designed Solidarity Trial monitors the effects of potential COVID-19 drug treatments in more than 14,000 participants across 52 countries (WHO, 2021a). While interim results found only corticosteroids to be effective at treating severe COVID-19, trials are still ongoing.

> *Conclusion 3-3: A priority for the development of seasonal and pandemic influenza vaccines in the dimension of clinical science is the design of surveillance activities that would support the demonstration of vaccine effectiveness and safety postauthorization.*

> *Conclusion 3-4: Population-based studies of VE also need to capture the racial/ethnic, socioeconomic, age, and medical conditions diversity within and across countries, in order to ensure confidence in vaccine effectiveness.*

> *Conclusion 3-5: To control for other variables that may bias VE, electronic medical records can be used to provide context on comorbidities that may affect VE, such as immunosuppression. Additional factors that may affect influenza vaccine VE include exposure risk, infection and vaccination history, and more indirect effects like herd immunity (Hollingsworth et al., 2021). These factors are more challenging to include in studies; their inclusion would allow better VE assessment and guide vaccine development.*

> *Conclusion 3-6: Existing networks collaborating to monitor influenza VE could be leveraged to provide the infrastructure to enable VE monitoring worldwide during a pandemic.*

Conclusion 3-7: An approach similar to the Solidarity Trial for COVID-19 treatments could provide opportunities to evaluate VE of multiple vaccine candidates simultaneously across a broad range of settings and populations (WHO, 2021a). Such international studies could support broad engagement, facilitate robust worldwide comparisons, and allow us to more quickly understand optimal use and allocation of vaccine candidates with differing profiles.

Postauthorization Vaccine Safety Surveillance

The COVID-19 pandemic has highlighted the critical role vaccine safety surveillance systems play in both detection of rare adverse events not identified in clinical trials and the effect of vaccine safety on decision making about use of vaccines in different countries. Some adverse events are so rare that they are not detected until millions of people have been vaccinated (Remmel, 2021). The ability to rapidly scale-up existing safety surveillance systems and implement novel approaches to surveillance is essential for real-time decision making during a pandemic.

Postmarket vaccine safety surveillance enables dynamic assessment of the benefit–risk balance. However, the assessment of benefit–risk balance may vary by country, as it depends on local burden of disease, type of populations prioritized, types of vaccines available for use, vaccine effectiveness of various vaccine candidates, values and preferences, and feasibility of implementation (Greenberg et al., 2016). Given the contextual variability, global benefit–risk assessments may not be useful to support uniform decision making.

Enhancing collaboration on vaccine safety is a critically important issue. Experience with COVID-19 vaccine safety highlights the need for such collaboration. For example, TTS was noted with the AstraZeneca COVID-19 vaccine in March 2021, which is an adenoviral vector vaccine (Meredith, 2021). In April 2021, the United States temporarily paused vaccination with the Janssen/J&J vaccine after six cases of TTS were identified, in part owing to similarities in the platform (Kupferschmidt and Vogel, 2021). In contrast, rare adverse events were detected more infrequently in LMICs, such as India that used many of the AstraZeneca vaccines for their population (Das and Mehta, 2021). On the other hand, data sharing increases the importance of data integrity, as incorrect information has the potential to spread further. One Canadian study showing excessive heart inflammation after COVID-19 vaccines was retracted after it was discovered to be a computation error (Miller, 2021). In addition, each vaccine safety surveillance system has unique strengths and limitations, particularly with regard to population coverage, types of vaccines used in these populations, timing of availability of vaccines for the population based on distribution efforts, and timing of availability of data for review and analysis. Standardization and harmonization between monitoring systems are essential for detecting rare adverse events and gathering accurate safety data (Li et al., 2021). Systems that can conduct signal evaluation activities in response to detected events are needed to support dynamic decision making about vaccine use (Remmel, 2021). Additional capabilities to support vaccine safety include the ability to generate background rates for rare events, to conduct rapid signal evaluations that incorporate chart validation, and to run formal epidemiologic studies to evaluate the risk of adverse events following vaccination in subpopulations. In the first two pandemic years, no vaccine-enhanced adverse reactions have been observed. However, what should happen and who should cover associated costs of such vaccine-associated events induced by novel COVID-19 or influenza vaccines is an area that should be explored in future reports.

Conclusion 3-8: As a core component of tailored benefit–risk assessments, countries need access to all available data relevant for decision making in their populations (WHO, 2019). Transparency in decision-making regarding key domains that influence recommendations for use and clear communication about the rationale for decisions is vital to support vaccine confidence, particularly if different decisions are made about authorization or use of vaccines in different countries.

Conclusion 3-9: Since postauthorization vaccine safety surveillance is crucial for vaccine confidence, timely and transparent vaccine communication may be just as important as the science and data on vaccine safety.

Conclusion 3-10: Harmonization between organizations is key. EMA and the European Centre for Disease Prevention and Control have initiated a program to jointly monitor postmarket safety monitoring and vaccine effectiveness (Balfour, 2021). WHO can play an important role in this, as its global advisory committee on vaccine safety, the Strategic Advisory Group of Experts, can make recommendations (WHO, 2021b).

RECOMMENDATIONS

Recommendation 3-1: The World Health Organization, in collaboration with national public health agencies (e.g., the U.S. Centers for Disease Control and Prevention, the European Centre for Disease Prevention and Control, the China Center for Disease Control and Prevention, and the Africa Centres for Disease Control and Prevention) should

conduct burden-of-disease studies in low- and middle-income countries to understand factors such as the health and economic burden of influenza illness and barriers to immunization in adult, pregnant, and pediatric populations to ensure development of infrastructure and capacity needed for pandemic vaccine development and implementation. Cost–benefit analyses should include additional economic productivity losses caused by delayed access to a vaccine in a pandemic.

Recommendation 3-2: The International Coalition of Medicines Regulatory Authorities and the World Health Organization, in partnership with national regulatory (e.g., the U.S. Food and Drug Administration and the European Medicines Agency) and public health agencies (e.g., the U.S. Centers for Disease Control and Prevention, the European Centre for Disease Prevention and Control, the China Center for Disease Control and Prevention, and the Africa Centres for Disease Control and Prevention) should invest, on a global level, in data infrastructure and capacity building to conduct real-time sentinel site surveillance of vaccine safety and effectiveness of different vaccine products deployed for use in epidemics and pandemics in diverse populations (e.g., age group, gender, race/ethnicity, geographic, presence of comorbidities, pregnancy, and socioeconomics), including a plan to ensure coordination, collaboration, and data sharing across these sentinel surveillance sites.

Recommendation 3-3: The International Coalition of Medicines Regulatory Authorities and the World Health Organization (Global Advisory Committee on Vaccine Safety) should ensure international coordination and collaboration on the timely and transparent review of vaccine safety data during epidemics and pandemics to support real-time decision making about the use of vaccines. Safety data should be made available to support country-level benefit–risk assessments, particularly for low- and middle-income countries relying on regional data from sentinel sites conducting safety surveillance.

REFERENCES

AJMC (*American Journal of Managed Care*) Staff. 2021a. A timeline of COVID-19 developments in 2020. *American Journal of Managed Care*. https://www.ajmc.com/view/a-timeline-of-covid19-developments-in-2020 (accessed October 19, 2021).

AJMC Staff. 2021b. A timeline of COVID-19 vaccine developments in 2021. *American Journal of Managed Care*. https://www.ajmc.com/view/a-timeline-of-covid-19-vaccine-developments-in-2021 (accessed October 19, 2021).

Alemayehu, C., G. Mitchell, and J. Nikles. 2018. Barriers for conducting clinical trials in developing countries—a systematic review. *International Journal for Equity in Health* 17(1):37. https://doi.org/10.1186/s12939-018-0748-6.

Balfour, H. 2021. EMA and ECDC to collaborate on post-marketing monitoring of COVID-19 vaccines. *European Pharmaceutical Review.* https://www.europeanpharmaceuticalreview.com/news/152318/ema-and-ecdc-to-collaborate-on-post-marketing-monitoring-of-covid-19-vaccines (accessed October 19, 2021).

Black, S. B., B. Law, R. T. Chen, C. L. Dekker, M. Sturkenboom, W.-T. Huang, M. Gurwith, and G. Poland. 2021. The critical role of background rates of possible adverse events in the assessment of COVID-19 vaccine safety. *Vaccine* 39(19):2712–2718. https://doi.org/10.1016/j.vaccine.2021.03.016.

Blumenthal, K. G., L. B. Robinson, C. A. Camargo Jr., E. S. Shenoy, A. Banerji, A. B. Landman, and P. Wickner. 2021. Acute allergic reactions to mRNA COVID-19 vaccines. *JAMA* 325(15):1562–1565. https://doi.org/10.1001/jama.2021.3976.

Bresee, J., J. Fitzner, H. Campbell, C. Cohen, V. Cozza, J. Jara, A. Krishnan, V. Lee, and the WHO Working Group on the Burden of Influenza Disease. 2018. Progress and remaining gaps in estimating the global disease burden of influenza. *Emerging Infectious Diseases* 24(7):1173–1177. https://doi.org/10.3201/eid2407.171270.

Brothers, W. 2020. *A timeline of COVID-19 vaccine development.* BioSpace. https://www.biospace.com/article/a-timeline-of-covid-19-vaccine-development (accessed October 19, 2021).

Buehler, J. W., R. S. Hopkins, J. M. Overhage, D. M. Sosin, and V. Tong. 2004. Framework for evaluating public health surveillance systems for early detection of outbreaks: Recommendations from the CDC Working Group. *MMWR Recommendations Report* 53(Rr-5):1–11.

Cashman, P., K. Macartney, G. Khandaker, C. King, M. Gold, and D. N. Durrheim. 2017. Participant-centred active surveillance of adverse events following immunisation: A narrative review. *International Health* 9(3):164–176. https://doi.org/10.1093/inthealth/ihx019.

CDC (U.S. Centers for Disease Control and Prevention). 2016. *Pregnant women and flu vaccination, Internet panel survey, United States, November 2016.* https://www.cdc.gov/flu/fluvaxview/pregnant-women-nov2016.htm (accessed October 19, 2021).

CDC. 2020. *Flu vaccination coverage, United States, 2019–20 influenza season.* https://www.cdc.gov/flu/fluvaxview/coverage-1920estimates.htm#:~:text=Results,-Children%20(6%20months&text=Among%20children%206%20months%20through%2017%20years%2C%20the%20percentage%20receiving,(62.6%25%3B%20Figure%201 (accessed October 19, 2021).

CDC. 2021a. *People with certain medical conditions.* https://www.cdc.gov/coronavirus/2019-ncov/need-extra-precautions/people-with-medical-conditions.html#:~:text=Similar%20to%20adults%2C%20children%20with,fully%20vaccinated%20against%20COVID%2D19 (accessed October 19, 2021).

CDC. 2021b. *V-safe.* https://www.cdc.gov/coronavirus/2019-ncov/vaccines/safety/vsafe.html (accessed October 19, 2021).

CDC. 2021c. *V-safe COVID-19 Vaccine Pregnancy Registry.* https://www.cdc.gov/coronavirus/2019-ncov/vaccines/safety/vsafepregnancyregistry.html (accessed October 19, 2021).

Chandler, R. E. 2020. Optimizing safety surveillance for COVID-19 vaccines. *Nature Reviews Immunology* 20(8):451–452. https://doi.org/10.1038/s41577-020-0372-8.

Collier, A. Y., K. McMahan, J. Yu, L. H. Tostanoski, R. Aguayo, J. Ansel, A. Chandrashekar, S. Patel, E. Apraku Bondzie, D. Sellers, J. Barrett, O. Sanborn, H. Wan, A. Chang, T. Anioke, J. Nkolola, C. Bradshaw, C. Jacob-Dolan, J. Feldman, M. Gebre, E. N. Borducchi, J. Liu, A. G. Schmidt, T. Suscovich, C. Linde, G. Alter, M. R. Hacker, and D. H. Barouch. 2021. Immunogenicity of COVID-19 mRNA Vaccines in pregnant and lactating women. *JAMA* 325(23):2370–2380. https://doi.org/10.1001/jama.2021.7563.

COMIT (COVID-19 Maternal Immunization Tracker). 2021. *COVID-19 vaccine policies on pregnancy*. https://www.comitglobal.org/pregnancy?policyPositions=1 (accessed October 19, 2021).

COVID Clinical Research Coalition. 2020. Global coalition to accelerate COVID-19 clinical research in resource-limited settings. *Lancet (London, England)* 395(10233):1322–1325. https://doi.org/10.1016/S0140-6736(20)30798-4.

Cunningham, E., and M. Iati. 2021. *Oxford pauses AstraZeneca vaccine trial in children*. https://www.washingtonpost.com/nation/2021/04/06/coronavirus-covid-live-updates-us (accessed October 19, 2021).

Das, K., and T. Mehta. 2021. India says "minuscule" clotting cases after AstraZeneca vaccine. *Reuters*. https://www.reuters.com/business/healthcare-pharmaceuticals/india-has-26-potential-cases-bleeding-clotting-after-astrazeneca-vaccine-2021-05-17 (accessed October 19, 2021).

Derhovanessian, E., and G. Pawelec. 2012. Vaccination in the elderly. *Microbial Biotechnology* 5(2):226–232. https://doi.org/10.1111/j.1751-7915.2011.00283.x.

Dooling, K., M. Marin, M. Wallace, N. McClung, M. Chamberland, G. M. Lee, H. K. Talbot, J. R. Romero, B. P. Bell, and S. E. Oliver. 2021. The Advisory Committee on Immunization Practices' Updated Interim Recommendation for Allocation of COVID-19 Vaccine—United States, December 2020. *Morbidity and Mortality Weekly Report* 69(5152):1657–1660. https://doi.org/10.15585/mmwr.mm695152e2.

EMA (European Medicines Agency). 2021a. *Conditional marketing authorisation*. https://www.ema.europa.eu/en/human-regulatory/marketing-authorisation/conditional-marketing-authorisation (accessed October 19, 2021).

EMA. 2021b. *COVID-19 vaccines: Development, evaluation, approval and monitoring*. https://www.ema.europa.eu/en/human-regulatory/overview/public-health-threats/coronavirus-disease-covid-19/treatments-vaccines/vaccines-covid-19/covid-19-vaccines-development-evaluation-approval-monitoring#monitoring-vaccine-safety-and-use-in-real-life-section (accessed October 19, 2021).

Excler, J.-L., M. Saville, S. Berkley, and J. H. Kim. 2021. Vaccine development for emerging infectious diseases. *Nature Medicine* 27(4):591–600.

FDA (U.S. Food and Drug Administration). 2021a. *Emergency Use Authorization for vaccines to prevent COVID-19*. https://www.fda.gov/media/142749/download (accessed October 19, 2021).

FDA. 2021b. COVID-19 vaccine safety surveillance. http://fda.gov/vaccines-blood-biologics/safety-availability-biologics/covid-19-vaccine-safety-surveillance (accessed October 19, 2021).

Feng, S., S. G. Sullivan, E. J. Tchetgen, and B. J. Cowling. 2021. The causal interpretation of "overall vaccine effectiveness" in test-negative studies. *American Journal of Epidemiology*. https://doi.org/10.1093/aje/kwab101.

Flores, L. E., W. R. Frontera, M. P. Andrasik, C. del Rio, A. Mondríguez-González, S. A. Price, E. M. Krantz, S. A. Pergam, and J. K. Silver. 2021. Assessment of the inclusion of racial/ethnic minority, female, and older individuals in vaccine clinical trials. *JAMA Network Open* 4(2):e2037640. https://doi.org/10.1001/jamanetworkopen.2020.37640.

Garg, S., L. Kim, M. Whitaker, A. O'Halloran, C. Cummings, R. Holstein, M. Prill, S. J. Chai, P. D. Kirley, N. B. Alden, B. Kawasaki, K. Yousey-Hindes, L. Niccolai, E. J. Anderson, K. P. Openo, A. Weigel, M. L. Monroe, P. Ryan, J. Henderson, S. Kim, K. Como-Sabetti, R. Lynfield, D. Sosin, S. Torres, A. Muse, N. M. Bennett, L. Billing, M. Sutton, N. West, W. Schaffner, H. K. Talbot, C. Aquino, A. George, A. Budd, L. Brammer, G. Langley, A. J. Hall, and A. Fry. 2020. Hospitalization rates and characteristics of patients hospitalized with laboratory-confirmed coronavirus disease 2019—COVID-NET, 14 States, March 1–30, 2020. *Morbidity and Mortality Weekly Report* 69(15):458–464. https://doi.org/10.15585/mmwr.mm6915e3.

Gee, J., P. Marquez, J. Su, G. M. Calvert, R. Liu, T. Myers, N. Nair, S. Martin, T. Clark, L. Markowitz, N. Lindsey, B. Zhang, C. Licata, A. Jazwa, M. Sotir, and T. Shimabukuro. 2021. First month of COVID-19 vaccine safety monitoring—United States, December 14, 2020–January 13, 2021. *Morbidity and Mortality Weekly Report* 70(8):283–288. https://doi.org/10.15585/mmwr.mm7008e3.

Greenberg, M., F. Simondon, and M. Saadatian-Elahi. 2016. Perspectives on benefit-risk decision-making in vaccinology: Conference report. *Human Vaccines & Immunotherapeutics* 12(1):176–181. https://doi.org/10.1080/21645515.2015.1075679.

Hall, S., L. Kaplow, Y. Sun, and T. Zulu Holt. 2021. "None are safe until all are safe": COVID-19 vaccine rollout in low- and middle-income countries. McKinsey & Company. https://www.mckinsey.com/industries/healthcare-systems-and-services/our-insights/none-are-safe-until-all-are-safe-covid-19-vaccine-rollout-in-low-and-middle-income-countries (accessed October 19, 2021).

Helfand, R., and S. Pal. 2021. *Global vaccine safety in a pandemic.* Global Advisory Committee on Vaccine Safety (GACVS), World Health Organization Pharmacovigilance Regulation and Safety Team.

Heyse, J. F., B. J. Kuter, M. J. Dallas, P. Heaton, and REST Study Team. 2008. Evaluating the safety of a rotavirus vaccine: the REST of the story. *Clinical Trials (London, England)* 5(2):131–139. https://doi.org/10.1177/1740774508090507.

Hodgson, S. H., K. Mansatta, G. Mallett, V. Harris, K. R. W. Emary, and A. J. Pollard. 2021. What defines an efficacious COVID-19 vaccine? A review of the challenges assessing the clinical efficacy of vaccines against SARS-CoV-2. *Lancet Infectious Diseases* 21(2):e26–e35. https://doi.org/10.1016/S1473-3099(20)30773-8.

Hollingsworth, R., C. El Guerche-Séblain, T. Tsai, Y. Vasiliev, S. Lee, H. Bright, and P. Barbosa. 2021. Assessment of the benefits of seasonal influenza vaccination: Elements of a framework to interpret estimates of vaccine effectiveness and support robust decision-making and communication. *Influenza and Other Respiratory Viruses* 15(1):164–174. https://doi.org/10.1111/irv.12786.

Jackson, L. A., M. L. Jackson, J. C. Nelson, K. M. Neuzil, and N. S. Weiss. 2006. Evidence of bias in estimates of influenza vaccine effectiveness in seniors. *International Journal of Epidemiology* 35(2):337–344. https://doi.org/10.1093/ije/dyi274.

Kim, H. W., E. R. Jenista, D. C. Wendell, C. F. Azevedo, M. J. Campbell, S. N. Darty, M. A. Parker, and R. J. Kim. 2021. Patients with acute myocarditis following mRNA COVID-19 vaccination. *JAMA Cardiology*. https://doi.org/10.1001/jamacardio.2021.2828.

Kraigsley, A. M., K. A. Moore, A. Bolster, M. Peters, D. Richardson, M. Arpey, M. Sonnenberger, M. McCarron, P. Lambach, H. C. Maltezou, and J. S. Bresee. 2021. Barriers and activities to implementing or expanding influenza vaccination programs in low- and middle-income countries: A global survey. *Vaccine* 39(25):3419–3427.

Kupferschmidt, K., and G. Vogel. 2021. Vaccine link to serious clotting disorder firms up. *Science* 372(6539):220. https://doi.org/10.1126/science.372.6539.220.

Lee, G. M., J. R. Romero, and B. P. Bell. 2020. Postapproval vaccine safety surveillance for COVID-19 vaccines in the US. *JAMA* 324(19):1937–1938. https://doi.org/10.1001/jama.2020.19692.

Li, X., A. Ostropolets, R. Makadia, A. Shoaibi, G. Rao, A. G. Sena, E. Martinez-Hernandez, A. Delmestri, K. Verhamme, P. R. Rijnbeek, T. Duarte-Salles, M. A. Suchard, P. B. Ryan, G. Hripcsak, and D. Prieto-Alhambra. 2021. Characterising the background incidence rates of adverse events of special interest for COVID-19 vaccines in eight countries: Multinational network cohort study. *BMJ* 373:n1435. https://doi.org/10.1136/bmj.n1435.

Mathioudakis, A. G., M. Ghrew, A. Ustianowski, S. Ahmad, R. Borrow, L. P. Papavasileiou, D. Petrakis, and N. D. Bakerly. 2021. Self-reported real-world safety and reactogenicity of COVID-19 vaccines: A vaccine recipient survey. *Life* 11(3):249. https://www.mdpi.com/2075-1729/11/3/249.

May, B. 2020. Moderna fully enrolls 30,000-person COVID-19 vaccine trial, boosts minority participation. BioSpace. https://www.biospace.com/article/moderna-fully-enrolls-30-000-person-covid-19-vaccine-trial-boosts-the-minority-study-population/ (accessed October 19, 2021).

Meredith, S. 2021. *More countries suspend AstraZeneca vaccinations over blood clot fears: What we know so far*. CNBC. https://www.cnbc.com/2021/03/12/astrazeneca-covid-vaccine-suspended-in-some-countries-over-blood-clot-fears.html (accessed October 19, 2021).

Miller, A. 2021. *A Canadian COVID-19 study that turned out to be wrong has spread like wildfire among anti-vaxxers*. CBC News. https://subscriptions.cbc.ca/newsletter_static/messages/secondopinion/2021-09-25 (accessed October 19, 2021).

Minnies, D., T. Hawkridge, W. Hanekom, R. Ehrlich, L. London, and G. Hussey. 2008. Evaluation of the quality of informed consent in a vaccine field trial in a developing country setting. *BMC Medical Ethics* 9(1):15. https://doi.org/10.1186/1472-6939-9-15.

NBAC (National Bioethics Advisory Commission). 2001. *Ethical and policy issues in international research: Clinical trials in developing countries*. Bethesda, MD: National Bioethics Advisory Commission.

Nsubuga, P., M. E. White, S. B. Thacker, M. A. Anderson, S. B. Blount, C. V. Broome, T. M. Chiller, V. Espitia, R. Imtiaz, D. Sosin, D. F. Stroup, R. V. Tauxe, M. Vijayaraghavan, and M. Trostle. 2006. Public health surveillance: A tool for targeting and monitoring interventions. In *Disease Control Priorities in Developing Countries*. Washington, DC: International Bank for Reconstruction, World Bank.

Ortiz, J. R., and K. M. Neuzil. 2019. Influenza immunization in low- and middle-income countries: Preparing for next-generation influenza vaccines. *Journal of Infectious Diseases* 219(Suppl 1):S97–S106. https://doi.org/10.1093/infdis/jiz024 (accessed October 19, 2021).

Pfizer. 2020. Pfizer and BioNTech conclude phase 3 study of COVID-19 vaccine candidate, meeting all primary efficacy endpoints. https://www.pfizer.com/news/press-release/press-release-detail/pfizer-and-biontech-conclude-phase-3-study-covid-19-vaccine (accessed October 19, 2021).

Rasmussen, S. A., D. J. Jamieson, and J. S. Bresee. 2008. Pandemic influenza and pregnant women. *Emerging Infectious Diseases* 14(1):95–100. https://doi.org/10.3201/eid1401.070667.

Razai, M. S., T. Osama, D. G. J. McKechnie, and A. Majeed. 2021. COVID-19 vaccine hesitancy among ethnic minority groups. *BMJ* 372:n513. https://doi.org/10.1136/bmj.n513.

Remmel, A. 2021. Why is it so hard to investigate the rare side effects of COVID vaccines? *Nature*. https://doi.org/10.1038/d41586-021-00880-9.

Ruf, B. R., and M. Knuf. 2014. The burden of seasonal and pandemic influenza in infants and children. *European Journal of Pediatrics* 173(3):265–276. https://doi.org/10.1007/s00431-013-2023-6.

Salmon, D. A., A. Akhtar, M. J. Mergler, K. S. Vannice, H. Izurieta, R. Ball, G. M. Lee, C. Vellozzi, P. Garman, F. Cunningham, B. Gellin, H. Koh, and N. Lurie. 2011. Immunization-safety monitoring systems for the 2009 H1N1 monovalent influenza vaccination program. *Pediatrics* 127(Suppl 1):S78–S86. https://doi.org/10.1542/peds.2010-1722L.

Sencer, D. J., and J. D. Millar. 2006. Reflections on the 1976 swine flu vaccination program. *Emerging Infectious Diseases* 12(1):29–33. https://doi.org/10.3201/eid1201.051007.

Shanes, E. D., S. Otero, L. B. Mithal, C. A. Mupanomunda, E. S. Miller, and J. A. Goldstein. 2021. Severe acute respiratory syndrome coronavirus 2 (SARS-CoV-2) vaccination in pregnancy: Measures of immunity and placental histopathology. *Obstetrics & Gynecology*. https://doi.org/10.1097/aog.0000000000004457.

Shimabukuro, T. T., S. Y. Kim, T. R. Myers, P. L. Moro, T. Oduyebo, L. Panagiotakopoulos, P. L. Marquez, C. K. Olson, R. Liu, K. T. Chang, S. R. Ellington, V. K. Burkel, A. N. Smoots, C. J. Green, C. Licata, B. C. Zhang, M. Alimchandani, A. Mba-Jonas, S. W. Martin, J. M. Gee, and D. M. Meaney-Delman. 2021. Preliminary findings of mRNA Covid-19 vaccine safety in pregnant persons. *New England Journal of Medicine* 384(24):2273–2282. https://doi.org/10.1056/NEJMoa2104983.

Soiza, R. L., C. Scicluna, and E. C. Thomson. 2021. Efficacy and safety of COVID-19 vaccines in older people. *Age and Ageing* 50(2):279–283. https://doi.org/10.1093/ageing/afaa274.

Sridhar, S., K. A. Brokstad, and R. J. Cox. 2015. Influenza vaccination strategies: Comparing inactivated and live attenuated influenza vaccines. *Vaccines* 3(2):373–389. https://doi.org/10.3390/vaccines3020373.

Standaert, B., T. Dort, J. Linden, A. Madan, S. Bart, L. Chu, M. S. Hayney, M. Kosinski, R. Kroll, J. Malak, G. Meier, N. Segall, and A. Schuind. 2019. Usability of daily SF36 questionnaires to capture the QALD variation experienced after vaccination with AS03A-adjuvanted monovalent influenza A (H5N1) vaccine in a safety and tolerability study. *Health and Quality of Life Outcomes* 17(1):80. https://doi.org/10.1186/s12955-019-1147-4.

Stuurman, A. L., T. Verstraeten, and A. De Schryver. 2017. Rapid assessment of the reactogenicity of a 2016-2017 seasonal influenza vaccine: Results from a feasibility study. *Expert Review of Vaccines* 16(2):187–191. https://doi.org/10.1080/14760584.2017.1264272.

Subbaraman, N. 2021. Pregnancy and COVID: What the data say. *Nature* 591(7849):193–195. https://doi.org/10.1038/d41586-021-00578-y.

Sullivan, S. G., S. Feng, and B. J. Cowling. 2014. Potential of the test-negative design for measuring influenza vaccine effectiveness: A systematic review. *Expert Review of Vaccines* 13(12):1571–1591. https://doi.org/10.1586/14760584.2014.966695.

Van Spall, H. G. C. 2021. Exclusion of pregnant and lactating women from COVID-19 vaccine trials: A missed opportunity. *European Heart Journal* ehab103.

Webb Hooper, M., A. M. Nápoles, and E. J. Pérez-Stable. 2020. COVID-19 and racial/ethnic disparities. *JAMA* 323(24):2466–2467. https://doi.org/10.1001/jama.2020.8598.

Wei, C.-J., M. C. Crank, J. Shiver, B. S. Graham, J. R. Mascola, and G. J. Nabel. 2020. Next-generation influenza vaccines: Opportunities and challenges. *Nature Reviews Drug Discovery* 19(4):239–252. https://doi.org/10.1038/s41573-019-0056-x.

Weir, J. P., and M. F. Gruber. 2016. An overview of the regulation of influenza vaccines in the United States. *Influenza and Other Respiratory Viruses* 10(5):354–360. https://doi.org/10.1111/irv.12383.

WHO (World Health Organization). 2019. *Global Vaccine Safety Blueprint 2.0 (GVSB2.0).* https://www.who.int/vaccine_safety/Draft_GVSB2.0_20190929.pdf?ua=1 (accessed October 19, 2021).

WHO. 2021a. *"Solidarity" clinical trial for COVID-19 treatments.* https://www.who.int/emergencies/diseases/novel-coronavirus-2019/global-research-on-novel-coronavirus-2019-ncov/solidarity-clinical-trial-for-covid-19-treatments (accessed October 19, 2021).

WHO. 2021b. *Strategic Advisory Group of Experts on Immunization (SAGE): About us.* https://www.who.int/groups/strategic-advisory-group-of-experts-on-immunization/about (accessed October 19, 2021).

Williams, S. R., A. J Driscoll, H. M. LeBuhn, W. H. Chen, K. M. Neuzil, and J. R. Ortiz. 2021. National routine adult immunisation programmes among World Health Organization member states: An assessment of health systems to deploy COVID-19 vaccines. *Eurosurveillance* 26(17):2001195.

Zanardi, L. R., P. Haber, G. T. Mootrey, M. T. Niu, and M. Wharton. 2001. Intussusception among recipients of rotavirus vaccine: Reports to the vaccine adverse event reporting system. *Pediatrics* 107(6):E97. https://doi.org/10.1542/peds.107.6.e97 (accessed October 19, 2021).

4

Manufacturing Science

The momentum created during the COVID-19 pandemic has highlighted the importance of speedy, high-quality, scalable, reliable, and affordable vaccine manufacturing, as means to prepare and respond quickly to potential influenza pandemics (Aars et al., 2021). Adding to the current influenza vaccine manufacturing landscape described in Chapter 1, understanding pandemic vaccine manufacturing preparedness and new vaccine technologies that have been rapidly developed and achieved first authorization during the COVID-19 pandemic offers the potential to be used for influenza pandemic preparedness (CEA, 2019). This chapter considers how to build on the momentum of the COVID-19 vaccines through continued progress on the strengthening of influenza vaccine manufacturing science and preparedness. The audacious goal would be to ensure that there is active global manufacturing capacity to produce up to 20 billion doses in 1 year to cover at least 80 percent of the world's population in the event of an influenza pandemic (Hoyt and Johnston, 2021).

This chapter addresses the third of the four dimensions of vaccine research, development, and manufacturing examined by the committee. It begins by describing the role of manufacturing science in the development of COVID-19 vaccines. The chapter then considers how lessons learned from the production of COVID-19 vaccines (shown in Box 4-1) can be applied to both seasonal and pandemic influenza vaccines in the dimension of manufacturing science. The final section presents recommendations drawn from these findings.

BOX 4-1
Manufacturing Science: Lessons Learned from the COVID-19 Pandemic

- Supply shortages, including laboratory reagents and materials, combined with inadequate manufacturing capacity caused significant delays in vaccine production.
- Unprecedented knowledge transfer and cost sharing between manufacturers allowed for the ability to scale-up and scale-out production capacity.
- The online publication of the SARS-CoV-2 genetic sequence allowed for rapid production of multiple vaccine candidates.
- Previous research and development (R&D) for zoonotic coronavirus vaccines (SARS-CoV, MERS-CoV) and lessons learned from pre-pandemic and pandemic influenza vaccine R&D was used to quickly advance the manufacturing science of COVID-19 vaccines.
- Because of vaccine nationalism, most of the vaccines first approved in North America and Europe were manufactured in and purchased by high-income countries (HICs), allowing distribution to HICs first.
- Lack of manufacturing capacity and vaccination programs in low- and middle-income countries (LMICs) significantly slowed vaccine rollout in those areas.
- Multi-agency collaborations can create programs such as COVAX that can help ensure equitable vaccine production in and distribution to LMICs.

MANUFACTURING SCIENCE AND THE DEVELOPMENT OF COVID-19 VACCINES

Global collaboration is essential during pre-pandemic and pandemic times. An increase in the number of vaccine manufacturers establishing new partnerships, collaborations, and agreements to adopt or strengthen manufacturing scale-up and scale-out capabilities has helped accelerate the fast rollout of the COVID-19 vaccines. In early 2020, manufacturers, as well as governments, began to invest in ramping up manufacturing capacity (scale-up) and establishing partnerships with other manufacturers (scale-out) to produce the needed supplies of COVID-19 vaccines (Hoyt and Johnston, 2021). Governments pledged billions of dollars to companies with promising candidates. For example, the U.S. government-initiated public–private partnership Operation Warp Speed invested more than $10 billion in the clinical development and manufacturing of COVID-19 vaccines (HHS, 2020b). There are limits to expanding capacity in the short term, and establishing new facilities is a time-consuming process. Still, the progress made in this regard during the COVID-19 pandemic points to the opportunity to improve global manufacturing capacity for influenza vaccines and set a course for sustainability and continued progress, including preparedness for pandemic influenza.

The development of COVID-19 vaccines has also highlighted the role of basic and translational research in accelerating vaccine development (see Chapter 2). The online publication of the viral sequence made a major difference in the development of vaccines against COVID-19. On January 10, 2020, the SARS-CoV-2 sequence was posted online (Paden et al., 2020), and laboratories worldwide used this sequence to design, synthesize, and develop COVID-19 vaccine candidates. The Global Initiative on Sharing All Influenza Data (GISAID) played an important role by providing a mechanism that both producers of sequence data and consumers of sequence data found mutually acceptable. It worked very well in this pandemic response, as it had worked during the 2013 pre-pandemic H7N9 influenza outbreak (Hay and McCauley, 2018). It took approximately 1 week to produce mRNA and DNA vaccine candidates from the published sequence, 3 weeks to produce viral vectors, and 2 months to produce protein-based candidates (Corbett et al., 2020; Rappuoli et al., 2021). Therefore, different platforms had very different development times during COVID-19, with the novel mRNA vaccine technology being the platform with the fastest development timelines to create a vaccine prototype.

Use of the various new production platforms used to manufacture COVID-19 vaccines also has illuminated the complexities of the vaccine development ecosystem and the many challenges that manufacturers face. For instance, supply shortages occurred during the COVID-19 response, in the manufacturing of not only the specific vaccines but also all laboratory reagents and materials (Rele, 2021). There were some specific, unanticipated challenges, such as an unanticipated pipette tip shortage (Woolston, 2021). Furthermore, there was a shortage in supply of specialty chemicals, such as some of the lipid components of lipid nanoparticles (Schmidt, 2021). Similar shortages have been observed in previous pandemic outbreaks of influenza, such as H1N1 in 2009, with respect to shortages of sterile eggs, cell lines, and other necessary tools.

International institutions and organizations played a critical role in the production of COVID-19 vaccines. The COVAX project was established between the World Health Organization (WHO); the Coalition for Epidemic Preparedness Innovations (CEPI); Gavi, the Vaccine Alliance; and the United Nations Children's Fund (UNICEF) for the distribution and procurement of COVID-19 vaccines. COVAX is part of the Access to COVID-19 Tools Accelerator that aims to guarantee a fair and equitable global access to vaccines (Gavi, 2021a). These sorts of multilateral collaborations can guarantee procurement of vaccines to ensure a sustainable market for any manufactured product. Gavi, the Vaccine Alliance now procures vaccines for 17 diseases and negotiates pricing for various regions, having lower-income countries contribute a lower share of the costs (Gavi, 2021b).

Beyond actual production of the COVID-19 vaccines, manufacturers increased capacity at early clinical trial stages to be ready to start distribution immediately after authorization. Additionally, various scale-out initiatives were undertaken where manufacturers agreed to produce vaccines developed by other companies. For example, Merck agreed to manufacture the Johnson & Johnson vaccine, while Sanofi and Novartis manufactured the Pfizer-BioNTech vaccine (Merck, 2021; Novartis, 2021; Sanofi, 2021). Increasingly, the pharmaceutical industry has outsourced manufacturing to contract manufacturing organizations, which can aid in reducing costs and, as such, lower the financial risk at an early stage of development. Furthermore, it would be useful if vaccine producers shared more data during the preclinical and clinical development of pandemic vaccinations. GISAID proved to be an exceptionally effective mechanism for sharing data of viral isolate sequences during the COVID-19 pandemic, providing a model for similar efforts to be made for other data.

During the COVID-19 pandemic, many pharmaceutical and vaccine companies have been generous and altruistic in sharing knowledge and costs and optimizing collaboration, but such collaboration is exceptional and may not become common practice or applicable during interpandemic periods (Knobler et al., 2020). Renewed business and financial strategies (short- and long-term) will be needed and are critical to ensuring a global, sustainable vaccine manufacturing framework, particularly in low- and middle-income countries (LMICs).

Finally, many of the COVID-19 vaccine candidates have involved a university or college assisting in preclinical research or clinical trials. For example, the AstraZeneca–University of Oxford vaccine started as a collaboration between the Jenner Institute of the University of Oxford and a spin-off company, Vaccitech (AstraZeneca, 2020a). Financing of development came from various sources, including Oxford Sciences Innovation, Google Ventures, and Sequoia Capital (Baker, 2020). To produce doses for the initial clinical trials, a collaboration was set up with the Italian company Advent Srl (IRBM Group, 2020), after which an agreement was signed between AstraZeneca, CEPI, and Gavi that secured the production of 300 million doses. An additional agreement was signed with the Serum Institute of India for 1 billion doses to be allocated to LMICs (AstraZeneca, 2020b). Similar collaborations existed for other vaccines, such as when Pfizer and Moderna teamed up to create an mRNA influenza vaccine (BioNTech, 2018).

MANUFACTURING SCIENCE: APPLYING LESSONS FROM THE PRODUCTION OF COVID-19 VACCINES TO VACCINES FOR INFLUENZA

Lessons learned from the production of COVID-19 vaccines highlight the critical importance of pandemic vaccine manufacturing preparedness, especially at the global level. Particular needs demonstrated by the COVID-19 experience include the establishment of (1) continuous, adaptive, flexible, and sustainable manufacturing infrastructure; (2) incentives to enable and facilitate strong, coordinated collaborations among manufacturers; and (3) establishment of global and local support manufacturing networks. In addition, given the vital role vaccine manufacturers play and their responsibilities and accountabilities for the products they develop, produce, and license, the committee identified specific actions that would strengthen seasonal and pandemic influenza vaccine manufacturing. The following sections detail lessons learned from the production of COVID-19 vaccines that can be applied to the manufacturing of influenza vaccines in the areas of global vaccine manufacturing preparedness, scientific and technical considerations, accelerating the timeline for vaccine production, the role of manufacturers and global manufacturing inequities, economic and market considerations, and global stakeholders and international collaborations.

Global Vaccine Manufacturing Preparedness

The 2019–2030 WHO Global Influenza Strategy, the 2020–2030 U.S. National Influenza Vaccine Modernization Strategy, and other documents stress the importance of optimizing global influenza vaccine manufacturing science and technology (HHS, 2020a; WHO, 2019). The COVID-19 pandemic has provided clarity on the need for a global effort to strengthen vaccine manufacturing capacity and response commensurate with the size of the global problem—a need highlighted above.

The speed at which a vaccine can be designed, developed, produced, tested, authorized, and widely and equitably distributed is the driving factor behind the response to a pandemic, significantly affecting the spread and burden of disease. A rapid response not only provides vital health benefits but also addresses important social and economic consequences (Shang et al., 2021). Therefore, considering the speed of developing a safe and effective vaccine is of the essence for pandemic influenza vaccine development and preparedness. Box 4-2 outlines transformations in vaccine research, development, and production applied to producing COVID-19 vaccines that helped accelerate manufacturing timelines.

Scientific and Technical Considerations

Pre-Pandemic Vaccines

For influenza, continuous monitoring systems for circulating influenza strains, such as the Tool for Influenza Pandemic Risk Assessment, developed by WHO in 2016, are very valuable for rapid identification of new virus strains that have the potential to cause a pandemic (Harrington et

BOX 4-2
Transformations in Vaccine Research, Development, and Production That Accelerated Manufacturing Timelines for COVID-19 Vaccines

- Information systems, data transfer and sharing
  - Online distribution of genetic information of viruses, instead of virus shipping, was critical for speedy COVID-19 vaccine development.
  - Information systems (Internet, artificial intelligence, data science) and open access data sharing (i.e., preprint servers) accelerate knowledge transfer, vaccine research and development, and sharing of vaccine pharmacovigilance data.
  - Collaborate with regulatory bodies to agree on requirements, enable rolling submission of data, and secure investments to manufacture vaccine prior to clinical trial results.
- New and novel vaccine technologies, processes, and evaluation
  - Digital-based (RNA, DNA) vaccine platforms have shorter development and production timelines compared to conventional whole inactivated virus and egg-based, cell-based, and protein-based platforms.
  - Innovative clinical trial designs enabled rapid assessment of vaccine products.

al., 2021). These strains can therefore be used to develop, manufacture, and stockpile so-called pre-pandemic vaccines. These vaccines would be deployed and used early in a pandemic response, diminishing the disease burden and allowing for pandemic-specific vaccines to be advanced in parallel. Currently, there are few pre-pandemic vaccines licensed for influenza (Soema et al., 2015). However, AUDENZ, an influenza A H5N1 adjuvanted monovalent vaccine, was approved by the U.S. Food and Drug Administration (FDA) in February 2020 and is the first of its kind designed to be stockpiled to protect against an influenza A pandemic (Cision PR Newswire, 2020).

Vaccine Platform Technologies

The years of research and development (R&D) for SARS-CoV and MERS-CoV vaccines offered an advantage to speed up the process and to rapidly advance manufacturing science for COVID-19. For instance, the discovery of di-proline mutation stabilization of pre-fusion S from MERS-CoV and the subsequent demonstration that this mutation also stabilized pre-fusion S from seasonal coronaviruses and SARS-CoV enabled the rapid adoption for SARS-CoV-2 vaccines (Duan et al., 2020; Pallesen et al., 2017). Prior work also permitted an acceleration of the vaccine products into clinical phases of development, with the time to start the first COVID-19 clinical trials approximately 66 days for mRNA vaccines, 3 months for viral vector vaccines, and 6 months for protein-based vaccines (Corbett et al., 2020; Rappuoli et al., 2021).

The seasonal influenza vaccine production process is a well-established machine that renews vaccines every 6 months. Every year, an estimated 1.48 billion doses of influenza vaccines can be produced and used for seasonal influenza programs worldwide. Despite the current infrastructure, however, an influenza pandemic may require rapid capability to manufacture 4.15–8.31 billion doses to produce and distribute a sufficient number of vaccine doses in a timely and equitable manner worldwide (Sparrow et al., 2021) (see Figure 4-1). The current vaccine production strategy for an influenza pandemic is to switch manufacturing capacity for seasonal vaccine into production of pandemic vaccines. Seasonal vaccines consist of multiple strains, so, for instance, the four-strain vaccine would translate into four doses of a single-strain pandemic vaccine, depending on the dose of the antigen or whether a dose-sparing adjuvant is included. In addition, the seasonal manufacturing is restricted to a time limit between the provision of seeds until a target number of doses is prepared for the season; a pandemic would not have such time restrictions. Approximately 90 percent of seasonal vaccines in use are inactivated virus vaccines (Matthews, 2006). Out of these, 90 percent are produced using the embryonated chicken egg-based platform (Bender, 2019).

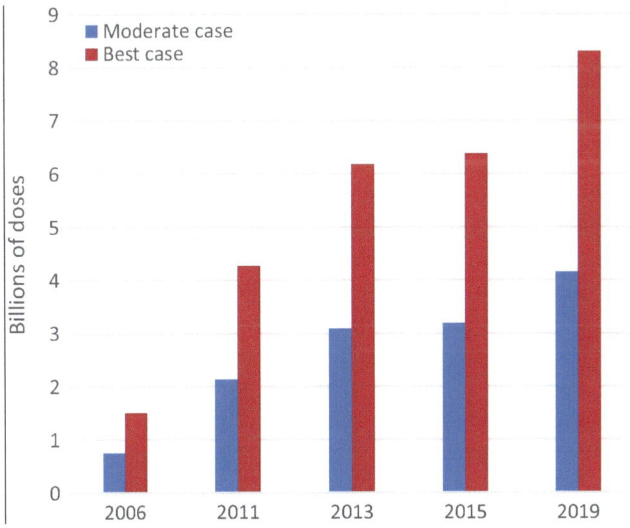

FIGURE 4-1 Estimated potential annual pandemic production capacity over time (since 2006).
SOURCE: Sparrow et al., 2021.

Reliance on the egg-based platform to meet the demands for pandemic vaccine production is challenging. First, to produce the large number of vaccines necessary during a pandemic, all seasonal vaccine manufacturing capacity must be converted to pandemic vaccine production at maximum capacity. Second, the time between strain selection and administering vaccines is lengthy as egg-based vaccine production averages 6 months (Rajaram et al., 2020). Third, production strategy is dependent on supplies. As noted earlier, during the COVID-19 pandemic, supply chain issues became a rate-limiting step due to increases in demand and reduced production and delivery of raw materials (Hatchett et al., 2021; Paris, 2020; Rele, 2021). Finally, the bottleneck for producing these vaccines is a steady supply of embryonated chicken eggs (Buckland, 2015). Therefore, investment in alternative platforms is necessary to ensure readiness for the next influenza pandemic.

> *Conclusion 4-1: A pandemic would require an increase in manufacturing facilities that would be cost-effective only if they were used beyond pandemic vaccine production (Plotkin et al., 2017). Therefore, public–private partnerships are needed to invest in this technology to produce vaccines for seasonal influenza to ensure preparedness for a pandemic.*

Cell-Based Technology

As discussed previously, the current principal alternative vaccine production platform uses cell-based technology (Rajaram et al., 2020). These vaccines are currently more expensive than vaccines produced using the egg-based system (Ng, 2012).

mRNA-Based Vaccines

The speedy development and high efficacy rate of mRNA-based vaccines for COVID-19 have fueled the attention and faith in the mRNA vaccine platform technology (Tenforde et al., 2021). This creates an opportunity to employ mRNA technology to develop and test vaccines for other viruses, such as influenza, and their use in acute outbreaks. Vaccines relying on mRNA technology have reached prominent levels during the COVID-19 pandemic, showing that this platform can be feasible and safe for the use in pandemics (Anand and Stahel, 2021). During a pandemic response, those who would benefit from technology transfer are the same groups who would have to find means of using existing facilities to produce the vaccine. Therefore, such capacity building and technology transfer is best done during interpandemic periods and has been proposed by the G20 as a way to close the global gaps in pandemic preparedness (G20, 2021).

Conclusion 4-2: The capacity to manufacture RNA vaccines needs to be expanded with a blueprint for the establishment of continuous, adaptive, flexible, and sustainable manufacturing infrastructure. Improvements also need to be made to vaccine formulations to improve aspects such as the cold chain requirements for mRNA vaccines (Crommelin et al., 2021).

A 2021 analysis by Public Citizen estimates that to produce 8 billion doses of the Moderna COVID-19 mRNA vaccine in 1 year would require at least 55 production lines set in 14 different facilities and with a total investment of at least $23 billion (Kis and Rizvi, 2021). This highlights the need for distributed manufacturing. Indeed, WHO, with the goal to expand the capacity of LMICs to produce COVID-19 vaccines, launched a request for expressions of interest to advance a vaccine transfer hub for the technology transfer of mRNA vaccines immediately (WHO, 2021a). A total of 19 manufacturers from more than a dozen countries in Africa, Asia, and Latin America responded. However, proprietary issues have not been resolved at this moment and may be a limiting factor in achieving these goals to increase global manufacturing capacity. Box 4-3 summarizes gaps and challenges for the use of mRNA-based vaccines as a tool for influenza preparedness.

BOX 4-3
Gaps and Challenges for the Use of mRNA-based Vaccines as a Tool for Influenza Preparedness

- Publicly available information on production capacity remains scarce and fragmented.
- Production capacity varies widely among vaccines and vaccine platforms (e.g., mRNA vaccine manufacturing capacity does not currently exist widely).
- Clinical research is needed to establish the potential for influenza mRNA vaccines.
- The private sector could be encouraged to develop mRNA technology but would require incentives and commitments to surpass cost barriers.
- Limited available commercial manufacturing capacity with the possibility of expansion is not evenly spread across vaccine makers.
- Needs remain for improved cold chain, stability, and delivery platforms:
  - Fill and finish is a major constraint in the rollout of vaccines (i.e., yields are established from bulk and are dependent of viral strain and platform; needs for low dead–volume needles/syringes; access/approval of adjuvants).
  - Clinical trials are rate limiting.
  - Vaccine needs change as outbreaks, epidemics, and pandemics evolve.
  - Intellectual property rights limit production in theory, but in practice the capacity, know-how, and availability of materials are limiting factors.

Conclusion 4-3: In addition to the insufficient manufacturing capacity for mRNA vaccines, clinical data on the efficacy of mRNA vaccines for various types of viruses, including influenza, are very limited. Therefore, to make decisions on whether mRNA technology should be developed for influenza vaccines, clinical data need to be expanded.

Recombinant Protein Vaccines

Recombinant protein vaccines are another platform of interest for the development of influenza vaccines. Various platforms can be used for the production of recombinant proteins. Using mammalian and insect cell culture systems results in high-quality proteins with the correct posttranslational modifications. However, because of proprietary obstacles, use of these cell lines is relatively costly (Barr et al., 2018). Bacterial systems, such as the use of *Escherichia coli* are less costly but result in incorrect folding of the full-length HA domain (Aguilar-Yáñez et al., 2010; DuBois et al., 2011). Yeast systems are also less costly than mammalian cell lines, but yeast require culture in low pH conditions, which may result in hyperglycosylation of the protein (Murugan et al., 2013; Saelens et al., 1999). A diverse portfolio of vaccine platforms is essential to achieve the manufacturing capacity that will be required during a pandemic, and protein-based vaccines are an essential tool to be used in a pandemic when there is an enormous need for vaccines. Furthermore, the development and use of appropriately selected adjuvants could reduce barriers and timelines by decreasing the amount of vaccine antigen required per dose or by broadening, or lengthening, the conferred protection, possibly allowing protection even with single-dose vaccination (Lemoine et al., 2021).

Accelerating the Timeline for Influenza Vaccine Production

Leveraging Experience with Seasonal Influenza Vaccines to Enhance Pandemic Preparedness

In an influenza pandemic, the vaccine manufacturing capacity will be based on the seasonal influenza vaccine production ecosystem and will be better prepared compared to COVID-19. The existing conventional production capacity for seasonal influenza vaccines is well poised to have a rapid changeover and can be converted to pandemic vaccine production relatively rapidly (Rockman et al., 2020). This is an advantage in preparing for a pandemic influenza scenario, contrary to what occurred with the COVID-19 pandemic, where the world was not vaccine ready even after having suffered from two prior zoonotic coronavirus epidemics.

Conclusion 4-4: Historical knowledge of manufacturing seasonal and pandemic influenza vaccines can be used to further strengthen pandemic influenza vaccine R&D and ensure a path toward accelerated production and testing timelines. Manufacturing steps, such as the validation of bulk manufacturing and scale-up production, should be able to occur more rapidly compared to the production of COVID-19 vaccines.

Ensuring Fill and Finish Capacity and the Availability of Raw Materials

The manufacturing of pandemic vaccines can be planned and performed accurately only after the bulk vaccine is produced, as this is largely based on the yield and growth of the virus in egg-based or cell-based systems. Filling of vials can start only after the yield is established, and the yield will depend on the viral strain and vaccine platform used. As dosing and final filling requirements remain unknown until clinical trial data are available (see below), clinical trials are the rate-limiting step in this process. At present, moreover, the United States has the fill and finish capacity for approximately 150 million vaccines, whereas in the event of a pandemic, an estimated 600 million would be needed (NASEM, 2019).

Conclusion 4-5: Capacity for fill and finish needs to be expanded and strengthened, alongside the availability of other consumables, such as needles and syringes. Also crucial is the availability of the raw materials, such as chicken eggs, needed to manufacture the vaccines. To enable speed and avoid limitations in bulk manufacturing, these raw materials need to be made available rapidly and in sufficient quantities.

Advancing Vaccine Candidates Through Clinical Development

Other factors that can improve and accelerate the development time of pandemic vaccines include changes to the framework used for advancing vaccine candidates through clinical development. For influenza, when a novel virus is identified, bulk vaccine is produced and the United States creates a stockpile. However, the system of surveillance and development differs from that of seasonal vaccines. Unlike seasonal vaccines, pre-pandemic vaccines first have to be shown to induce immunogenicity in relevant populations, after which the vaccines need to undergo clinical trials to assess efficacy and safety before they are authorized for use in a pandemic. Such trials can, however, only be conducted once a pandemic is in progress. Traditionally, and before the COVID-19 pandemic, clinical phases I, II, and III of development generally occurred sequentially. During the COVID-19 pandemic, it became clear that these processes can be shortened by ensuring a seamless transition between clinical phases (GAO, 2021).

Investing in the Development of Platforms for Seasonal Influenza Vaccines

Continuous investments by the public sector are needed to develop a variety of vaccine platforms for seasonal influenza, including novel platforms such as mRNA and recombinant protein vaccines. Expansion of vaccine platforms will be gradual as the private sector develops the means to build capacity for novel vaccine development. During this period of capacity building, existing vaccine platforms will be important to meet the demand.

> *Conclusion 4-6: As digital technologies, the science of vaccine formulation, and adjuvant technologies expand, new platforms for the development of seasonal influenza vaccines will be needed to complement rather than replace conventional vaccine platforms.*

The Role of Manufacturers and Global Manufacturing Inequities

As discussed earlier, vaccine manufacturers have undergone significant transformation during the COVID-19 pandemic, and acceleration in technology transfer has been evident. However, global inequity in vaccine manufacturing and distribution continues to be a hurdle. As of 2019, there were 40 active influenza vaccine production facilities worldwide. Twenty of these were located in high-income countries (HICs), with 15 in upper-middle- and five in lower-middle-income countries (Sparrow et al., 2021). Box 4-4 lists the essential responsibilities of vaccine manufacturers, while Box 4-5 outlines the attributes of effective vaccine manufacturing technology transfer during pandemics.

Generally, vaccines are manufactured in HICs, and this affects distribution as these countries are also the first to receive vaccines and provide them to their population, while LMICs have minimal influenza vaccine manufacturing capacity (Palache et al., 2017). As of June 2021, one-third of HIC populations had received at least one dose of COVID-19 vaccine, compared to just 1 percent in LMICs (Berkley, 2021). As of September 2021, that percentage had only risen to just over 2 percent (Our World in Data, 2021) (see also Chapter 3). Many of these countries additionally have limited use of the seasonal influenza vaccines, as programs needed for that purpose are not in place. In some cases, this is due to the high costs of a vaccination program, while in other cases, it is caused by a need for surveillance to evaluate the need for a yearly program, competing demands, or the need

BOX 4-4
Essential Responsibilities and Functions of Manufacturers

- Efficiently produce vaccines that are purchased at a sustainable price, while meeting rigorous quality standards.
- Participate in research and development of vaccine technologies and manufacturing improvements.
- Quickly adapt to pandemic demands and supply chain changes.
- Share data.
- Participate in technology transfer, including technology adaptation and training activities with international partners.

BOX 4-5
Attributes of Effective Manufacturing Technology Transfer During Pandemics

- Adaptability and resilience
- Supply chain risk reduction
- Quality and safety practices
- Viability and design: assessment and infrastructure to receive new technologies
- Collaboration and information sharing
- Governance
- Communication
- Funding

to strengthen health systems (Sparrow et al., 2021). Consequently, it is important to overcome the obstacle of convincing certain regions of the world about the importance of investing in the seasonal influenza landscape, and even more so investing in the new vaccine platforms for influenza preparedness. This situation is complicated by the fact that the seasonal influenza vaccine has limited and variable efficacy and the fact that many LMICs lack the resources to make diagnoses and to identify new, rare adverse event patterns. Quality control, quality management, and pharmacovigilance are key factors contributing to past successes of technology transfer efforts and are essential for technology transfer to LMICs. Figures 4-2 and 4-3 show the prevalence of adult immunization programs in the world and reflect that many countries have influenza programs in place, particularly in Europe and the Americas. However, there appears to be a significant disparity in the existence of these programs between HICs and LMICs.

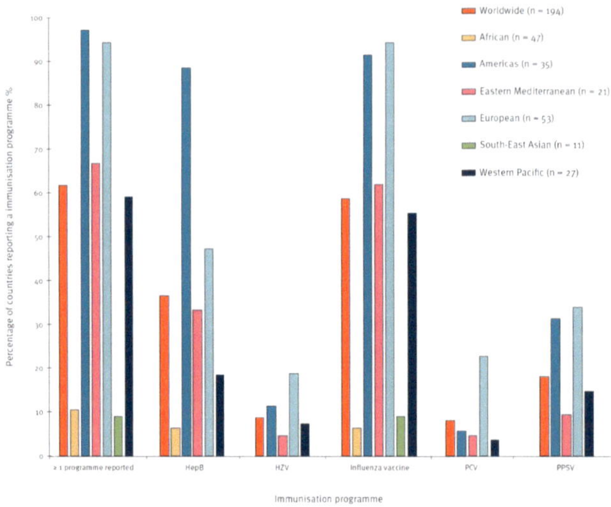

FIGURE 4-2 Countries reporting adult immunization programs by vaccine type and WHO region.
NOTE: Vaccines include Hepatitis B (HepB); Herpes Zoster (HZV), also known as Shingles; Influenza; Pneumococcal Conjugate (PCV); and Pneumococcal polysaccharide (PPSV).
SOURCE: Williams et al., 2021.

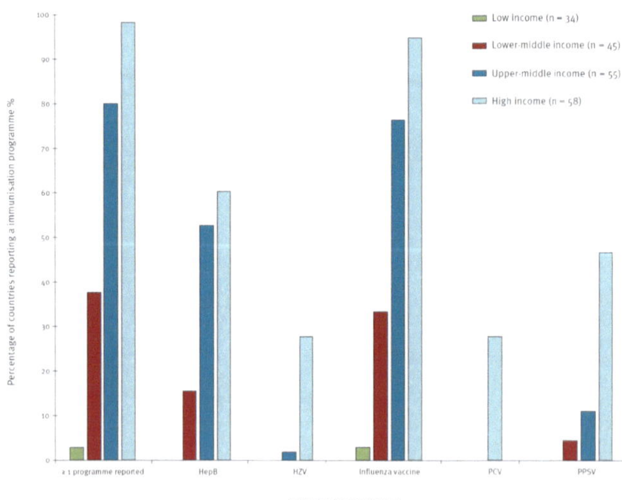

FIGURE 4-3 Countries reporting adult immunization programs by vaccine type and income level.
NOTE: Vaccines include Hepatitis B (HepB); Herpes Zoster (HZV), also known as Shingles; Influenza; Pneumococcal Conjugate (PCV); and Pneumococcal polysaccharide (PPSV).
SOURCE: Williams et al., 2021.

While LMICs currently lack the infrastructure for adequate vaccine manufacturing capacity (Figueroa et al., 2021), some initiatives to fill this gap have been conducted. In 2006, WHO launched the Global Action Plan (GAP) for influenza vaccines, intended to address predicted shortages of global vaccine supply when there is an influenza pandemic (Palkonyay and Fatima, 2016). Between 2009 and 2019, PATH supported vaccine manufacturers in Brazil, China, India, and other countries to develop, manufacture, and supply seasonal and pandemic influenza vaccines. The focus of these initiatives was on increasing capacity for both seasonal and pandemic vaccines, and thereby access to the vaccines in LMICs (PATH, 2019).

As noted earlier, during the COVID-19 pandemic, there were unprecedented partnerships between vaccine developers, which allowed the scale-up and scale-out of vaccine manufacturing in parallel with clinical development. Previous work was valuable in developing a model for accelerated vaccine development for COVID-19. Manufacturers have predicted the ability to produce 12 billion COVID-19 vaccines in 2021, which would be enough to vaccinate 70 percent of the world's population, assuming the majority would require two doses of vaccine (Irwin, 2021). However, since the moment the vaccines received Emergency Use Authorization in various countries, purchases by local governments have determined where the vaccines were distributed, resulting in vaccine inequity globally (Hyder et al., 2021). There is considerable variation in production capacity (see Figure 4-4) for various vaccine platforms, and not all vaccine producers can expand capacity evenly (Grand View Research, 2020). This makes it difficult for policy and decision makers to understand the supply chains involved and take urgent action where it is most required.

Additionally, global needs change continuously during a pandemic. This has also become evident during the COVID-19 pandemic. For instance, the emergence of virus variants of concern may require new vaccines or boosters, the length of immunity and need for boosters to extend immunity remains unknown, and it remains unclear whether and when the vaccines can be used for young children (WHO, 2021b). Additionally, some countries may want to purchase and store a surplus of vaccines for potential future use. These factors affect the requirements and the supply of vaccines to various regions of the world.

During a pandemic, manufacturers are generally more willing to collaborate than between pandemics. An example of a collaboration between manufacturers that has been initiated during the COVID-19 pandemic to scale-up and scale-out is the collaboration between AstraZeneca and the University of Oxford, each of which also has many partners for fill and finish (AstraZeneca, 2020a). Pfizer and BioNTech are an example of a successful alliance that allows novel technology developments from biotechnology companies to be developed at a large scale (Pfizer, 2020). Further collabora-

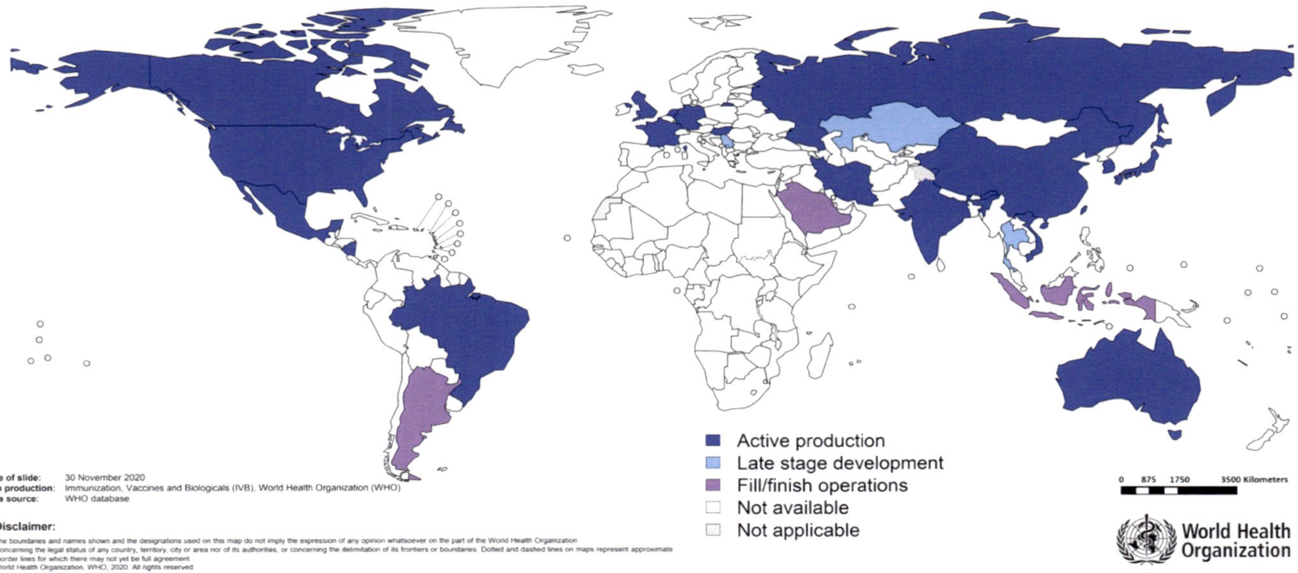

FIGURE 4-4 Countries with influenza vaccine production capacity in 2019.
SOURCE: Sparrow et al., 2021.

tion and technology transfer might enhance the global supply and lift the burden of the pandemic. However, technology transfer is not a matter of just handing over protocols. It is a complex process; training people and setting up a new facility with all the critical quality attributes, critical process parameters, and comparable protocols is a time-consuming and costly process. New facilities will have to set up supply chains, train people, and provide registration documentation to regulatory agencies. As an example, the Pfizer BioNTech collaboration started in August 2018 when the two companies began collaborating on an mRNA influenza vaccine (BioNTech, 2018). This allowed the companies to work together for a substantial period of time that was essential for the effective collaboration during the pandemic. Given the complexity and challenges of carrying out technology transfer with limited resources, an initiative was undertaken by WHO in 2007 in collaboration with the Netherlands Vaccine Institute to increase technology transfer of seasonal influenza vaccine manufacturing using the egg-based platform. The initiative included setting up a facility training hub built at an industrial scale for LMICs; 15 countries participated and received training and technical assistance (Hendriks et al., 2011). The program resulted in an expansion of the global manufacturing capacity for seasonal and pandemic influenza vaccines, but it also showed that long-term investments and local, national, and international regulatory agility, alignment, and consistency are critical, with seasonal influenza vaccine uptake locally as an essential factor.

Currently, then, there is a need to increase vaccine manufacturing capacity to strengthen global health security, as this capacity is the bottleneck in the current rollout of COVID-19 vaccines. To this end, a global manufacturing network is needed to build up regional infrastructure and expertise. In particular, the manufacturing structure requires collaborations for technical support or knowledge transfer; savvy management of intellectual property; methods for handling complexities in supply chains infrastructure; regulatory science (see Chapter 5); and robust financing to support the costs associated with preparedness and pandemic response (Aars et al., 2021; Hotez et al., 2021).

Conclusion 4-7: Global manufacturing networks can aid in establishing public–private partnerships to allow surge capacity in a pandemic. They can also help build up regional infrastructure and expertise in LMICs to expand manufacturing capacity in these regions and improve health security for the countries. There is a need for sustainable and transparent partnerships to make technology transfer successful and increase existing vaccine manufacturing capacity.

Chapter 2 emphasizes the importance of standardizing assays, reagents, and animal models for each vaccine platform. Technology transfer needs to include these standardized methods and high-quality data. Sustained funding for these developments from the public sector, in close collaboration with the private sector, is warranted, with the requirement that the private sector support the technology transfer.

Conclusion 4-8: To increase vaccine manufacturing globally, manufacturing processes need to be developed and facilities operationalized in LMICs. Vaccine manufacturing capacity in LMICs could be improved by enhancing technical competencies and quality management systems, providing technical support for the development of seasonal and pandemic influenza vaccines, and developing platforms for local technical training. These measures would help LMICs acquire the manufacturing knowledge needed to expand global production capacity.

Conclusion 4-9: LMICs also need support in the clinical development of newly manufactured vaccines to aid in coordinating and evaluating results of clinical trials. Additionally, given that manufacturers are responsible for safety, effectiveness, and product quality, their regulatory and pharmacovigilance capacity needs to be strengthened.

Conclusion 4-10: Considerable and continuous investment is necessary to establish manufacturing capacity in LMICs to prepare for a pandemic. Early involvement of key stakeholders, such as ministries of health, in the development of guidelines for the use of influenza vaccines is crucial. The socioeconomic costs of pandemics make these types of investments worthwhile. It will be essential to form regional manufacturing hubs of sufficient scale that are sustainable to meet the demands of a pandemic response. Local facilities focused on flexible fill and finish could also expand availability while reducing long-term costs and risks. Incentives will need to be provided regionally to ensure that there is a sustainable market for these vaccines.

Economic and Market Considerations

As discussed earlier, rapid advancement of COVID-19 vaccines, especially for mRNA-based platforms, was enabled by investments from the public sector into basic research contributing to establishing the mRNA vaccine technology and investments by the private sector, where shareholders took a financial risk of pandemic mRNA vaccine development and manufacturing. At the same time, the public sector provided the market for sales of the vaccine. Substantial and immediate investment in advanced vaccine manufacturing in parallel with investment in vaccine R&D is crucial to accelerating the manufacturing process. Distinguishing between highly effective forms of public expenditure—supporting the basic scientific research enterprise, maintaining intellectual property mechanisms that encourage private investment, and creating markets for pandemic vaccines—and forms of public expenditure with more mixed track records can help ensure the most effective future expenditures of public funds for pandemic preparedness. There is a particular need for public funds to address market failures, such as the timely supply of pandemic vaccine to LMICs. Additionally, the economic viability of manufacturing facilities, especially in LMICs, during interpandemic periods needs to be addressed; otherwise the investments in these facilities could fail.

For influenza vaccines, however, there would be a significant cost barrier to developing new and novel vaccines, considering egg-based vaccines are currently a far less expensive option (Chen et al., 2020). Moreover, barriers to entry, such as FDA licensing and regulatory requirements for vaccine manufacturers, make it difficult for new actors to enter the market (Honeycutt et al., 2005). To overcome these challenges, financial investments from the public and private sectors need to be ramped up and consolidated. For instance, there is interest among private companies, such as Pfizer and Moderna, in developing mRNA vaccines directed at influenza, which was in development pre-COVID-19, and the influenza vaccine research facilitated the COVID-19 vaccine response (Moderna, 2021; Pfizer, 2021).

A conflict that remains for these new vaccine manufacturing platforms is that the question of waiving intellectual property (IP) rights has not been settled (CGD, 2021). Several potential solutions have been proposed, including patent pools (Billette de Villemeur et al., 2021; Hotez et al., 2021). There are major cost differences between the various vaccine platforms, which are defined by the material IP, as some of these vaccine platforms are relatively new and there are some proprietary issues (Krishtel and Malpani, 2021; Martin and Lowery, 2020). There are also the costs of the infrastructure needed to create the ability to manufacture these types of vaccines (Excler et al., 2021; Rosa et al., 2021). However, IP protections were key factors that supported that development of the technologies and created the willingness of the private sector to invest in COVID-19 vaccines, including mRNA-based vaccines. There is a risk of counterproductive changes to the IP system when it comes to pandemic preparedness.

Volatile political climates have led to changes in the quality of R&D, manufacturing, and investments in vaccines (Califf et al., 2020). These changes in political environments and support can disrupt the global governance of the vaccine ecosystem, leading to changes in vaccine quality requirements, varied investment commitments, and inequality in the access and distribution of vaccines and the use and acceptance of vaccines. It is essential that appropriate value propositions be designed to justify investments in vaccination research, development, and manufacturing capacity extending beyond public health benefits to include the pandemic's major social and economic costs. The International Monetary Fund estimated the global economy lost $12 trillion in 2020–2021 as a result of the COVID-19 pandemic, a cost that could have been significantly offset with better vaccine preparedness (Academy Health, 2020).

> *Conclusion 4-11: Financial institutions, in conjunction with multilateral donors and private philanthropic organizations, need to recognize the potential public health and economic impacts of an influenza pandemic, hence incentivizing them to create sustainable financial vehicles and encouraging the financing of manufacturing organizations in LMICs. These investments will need to be sustained both for seasonal and pandemic influenza vaccine R&D activities and for the harmonization and mutual recognition of data and standards, equivalence agreements and quality control measures, and strengthening of regulatory and pharmacovigilance capacity.*

Global Stakeholders, International Collaborations, and Networks

As recently as 2005, the influenza vaccine market consisted of only two major manufacturers and was of little interest to new actors. It took the H5N1 outbreak of the same year for the United States and other stakeholders to expand the market, largely through public–private partnerships. These partnerships allowed new products to be developed, new manufacturers to enter the market, and production capacity to expand (Neal et al., 2020). Experience with the H5N1 influenza outbreak of 2005 and the COVID-19 pandemic can be used to guide preparation for the next influenza pandemic.

The COVID-19 vaccine development experience has highlighted shifts in the roles of different actors that engage during the vaccine development process. Vaccine partnerships between developers and manufacturers to perform scale-up and scale-out in parallel with clinical development are essential. The scientific community has called for a primer for change whereby, in addition to multi-national corporations, the academic sector, small biotech companies, and the entrance of developing country manufacturers would play more prominent roles in developing, testing, and supplying vaccines for the global markets (Aars et al., 2021).

> *Conclusion 4-12: International collaborations and global stakeholders are essential components of ensuring support for manufacturing science. An important consideration is to ensure that global and local*

manufacturing support networks exist and that the private sector is encouraged to participate in the development of manufacturing technologies. This requires providing incentives to enable and facilitate stronger, coordinated collaborations among manufacturers, primarily through contracts and commitments.

RECOMMENDATIONS

Recommendation 4-1: The U.S. Department of Health and Human Services and the World Health Organization should develop a plan for a sufficient and self-sustainable global supply of influenza vaccines for pandemics. This includes

- Convening, supporting, and encouraging multi-national, public, and private vaccine manufacturers to benchmark, prioritize, and harmonize influenza vaccine manufacturing; and
- Enhancing and expanding support of the global influenza vaccine manufacturing network, creating manufacturing hubs for greater collaboration, and building capacity to address challenges in manufacturing in low- and middle-income countries.

Recommendation 4-2: Vaccine manufacturers should take a risk-based approach to pandemic influenza preparedness. This approach would be most effective if incentivized, and could include

- Participating during research and development, data sharing, technology adoption, and training activities with international partners;
- Expanding internal capacity to assess the production needs and their risks;
- Using scientific evidence to design strategies to reduce risks (e.g., World Health Organization prequalification, licensing, and marketing); and
- Formalizing technology transfer (scale-up and scale-out) activities, taking into consideration timelines and the outcomes for equitable costs, access, and distribution.

REFERENCES

Aars, O. K., M. Clark, and N. Schwalbe. 2021. Increasing efficiency in vaccine production: A primer for change. *Vaccine: X* 8:100104.

AcademyHealth. 2020. *Research insights: The economics of vaccine development and supply: Responding to COVID-19 and preparing for the next threat.* https://academyhealth.org/sites/default/files/ah_ri_economics_of_vaccines_brief_final.pdf (accessed October 19, 2021).

Aguilar-Yáñez, J. M., R. Portillo-Lara, G. I. Mendoza-Ochoa, S. A. García-Echauri, F. López-Pacheco, D. Bulnes-Abundis, J. Salgado-Gallegos, I. M. Lara-Mayorga, Y. Webb-Vargas, F. O. León-Angel, R. E. Rivero-Aranda, Y. Oropeza-Almazán, G. M. Ruiz-Palacios, M. I. Zertuche-Guerra, R. M. DuBois, S. W. White, S. Schultz-Cherry, C. J. Russell, and M. M. Alvarez. 2010. An influenza A/H1N1/2009 hemagglutinin vaccine produced in *Escherichia coli*. *PLOS ONE* 5(7):e11694.

Anand, P., and V. P. Stahel. 2021. The safety of COVID-19 mRNA vaccines: A review. *Patient Safety in Surgery* 15(1):20.

AstraZeneca. 2020a. *AstraZeneca and Oxford University announce landmark agreement for COVID-19 vaccine*. https://www.astrazeneca.com/media-centre/press-releases/2020/astrazeneca-and-oxford-university-announce-landmark-agreement-for-covid-19-vaccine.html (accessed October 19, 2021).

AstraZeneca. 2020b. *AstraZeneca takes next steps towards broad and equitable access to Oxford University's potential COVID-19 vaccine*. Cambridge, UK: AstraZeneca.

Baker, S. 2020. COVID vaccine front-runner is months ahead of her competition. *Bloomberg Businessweek*. July 14.

Barr, I. G., R. O. Donis, J. M. Katz, J. W. McCauley, T. Odagiri, H. Trusheim, T. F. Tsai, and D. E. Wentworth. 2018. Cell culture-derived influenza vaccines in the severe 2017–2018 epidemic season: A step towards improved influenza vaccine effectiveness. *NPJ Vaccines* 3:44.

Bender, E. 2019. Accelerating flu protection. *Nature* 573(7774):S60–S61.

Berkley, S. 2021. Why we must improve vaccine manufacturing before the next pandemic. *TIME*. June 9.

Billette de Villemeur, E., V. Dequiedt, and B. Versaevel. 2021. Pool patents to get COVID vaccines and drugs to all. *Nature* 591(7851):529.

BioNTech. 2018. *BioNTech signs collaboration agreement with Pfizer to develop mRNA-based vaccines for prevention of influenza*. Mainz, Germany: BioNTech. August 16, 2018.

Buckland, B. C. 2015. The development and manufacture of influenza vaccines. *Human Vaccines & Immunotherapeutics* 11(6):1357–1360.

Califf, R., S. Gottlieb, M. Hamburg, J. Henney, D. Kessler, M. McClellan, and A. von Eschenbach. 2020. 7 former FDA commissioners: The Trump administration is undermining the credibility of the FDA. *The Washington Post*. October 2.

CEA (Council of Economic Advisers). 2019. *Mitigating the impact of pandemic influenza through vaccine innovation*. Washington, DC: White House.

CGD (Center for Global Development). 2021. *Would exempting COVID-19 vaccines from intellectual property rights improve global access and equity?* https://www.cgdev.org/debate/would-exempting-covid-19-vaccines-intellectual-property-rights-improve-global-access (accessed October 19, 2021).

Chen, J.-R., Y.-M. Liu, Y.-C. Tseng, and C. Ma. 2020. Better influenza vaccines: An industry perspective. *Journal of Biomedical Science* 27(1):33.

Cision PR Newswire. 2020. *Seqirus announces U.S. FDA approval of its first-ever adjuvanted, cell-based pandemic influenza a (h5n1) vaccine*. https://www.prnewswire.com/news-releases/seqirus-announces-us-fda-approval-of-its-first-ever-adjuvanted-cell-based-pandemic-influenza-a-h5n1-vaccine-300997595.html?tc=eml_cleartime (accessed October 19, 2021).

Corbett, K. S., D. Edwards, S. R. Leist, O. M. Abiona, S. Boyoglu-Barnum, R. A. Gillespie, S. Himansu, A. Schäfer, C. T. Ziwawo, A. T. DiPiazza, K. H. Dinnon, S. M. Elbashir, C. A. Shaw, A. Woods, E. J. Fritch, D. R. Martinez, K. W. Bock, M. Minai, B. M. Nagata, G. B. Hutchinson, K. Bahl, D. Garcia-Dominguez, L. Ma, I. Renzi, W.-P. Kong, S. D. Schmidt, L. Wang, Y. Zhang, L. J. Stevens, E. Phung, L. A. Chang, R. J. Loomis, N. E. Altaras, E. Narayanan, M. Metkar, V. Presnyak, C. Liu, M. K. Louder, W. Shi, K. Leung, E. S. Yang,

A. West, K. L. Gully, N. Wang, D. Wrapp, N. A. Doria-Rose, G. Stewart-Jones, H. Bennett, M. C. Nason, T. J. Ruckwardt, J. S. McLellan, M. R. Denison, J. D. Chappell, I. N. Moore, K. M. Morabito, J. R. Mascola, R. S. Baric, A. Carfi, and B. S. Graham. 2020. SARS-CoV-2 mRNA vaccine development enabled by prototype pathogen preparedness. *bioRxiv* 2020.2006.2011.145920.

Crommelin, D. J. A., T. J. Anchordoquy, D. B. Volkin, W. Jiskoot, and E. Mastrobattista. 2021. Addressing the cold reality of mRNA vaccine stability. *Journal of Pharmaceutical Sciences* 110(3):997–1001.

Duan, L., Q. Zheng, H. Zhang, Y. Niu, Y. Lou, and H. Wang. 2020. The SARS-CoV-2 spike glycoprotein biosynthesis, structure, function, and antigenicity: Implications for the design of spike-based vaccine immunogens. *Frontiers in Immunology* 11(2593).

DuBois, R. M., J. M. Aguilar-Yañez, G. I. Mendoza-Ochoa, Y. Oropeza-Almazán, S. Schultz-Cherry, M. M. Alvarez, S. W. White, and C. J. Russell. 2011. The receptor-binding domain of influenza virus hemagglutinin produced in escherichia coli folds into its native, immunogenic structure. *Journal of Virology* 85(2):865–872.

Excler, J.-L., M. Saville, S. Berkley, and J. H. Kim. 2021. Vaccine development for emerging infectious diseases. *Nature Medicine* 27(4):591–600.

Figueroa, J. P., M. E. Bottazzi, P. Hotez, C. Batista, O. Ergonul, S. Gilbert, M. Gursel, M. Hassanain, J. H. Kim, B. Lall, H. Larson, D. Naniche, T. Sheahan, S. Shoham, A. Wilder-Smith, N. Strub-Wourgaft, P. Yadav, and G. Kang. 2021. Urgent needs of low-income and middle-income countries for COVID-19 vaccines and therapeutics. *Lancet* 397(10274):562–564.

G20 (G20 High-Level Independent Panel). 2021. *A global deal for our pandemic age.* https://pandemic-financing.org/wp-content/uploads/2021/07/Four-Major-Gaps.pdf (accessed October 19, 2021).

GAO (U.S. Government Accountability Office). 2021. *Operation Warp Speed: Accelerated COVID-19 vaccine development status and efforts to address manufacturing challenges.* https://www.gao.gov/products/gao-21-319 (accessed October 19, 2021).

Gavi (The Vaccine Alliance). 2021a. *COVAX.* https://www.gavi.org/covax-facility (accessed October 19, 2021).

Gavi. 2021b. *Facts and figures.* https://www.gavi.org/programmes-impact/our-impact/facts-and-figures (accessed October 19, 2021).

Grand View Research. 2020. *COVID-19 vaccines market production capacity & development timeline: (by type: Virus-like particle (VLP), whole virus, protein, antibodies, viral vector, mRNA/DNA).* https://www.grandviewresearch.com/industry-analysis/covid-19-vaccines-market (accessed October 19, 2021).

Harrington, W. N., C. M. Kackos, and R. J. Webby. 2021. The evolution and future of influenza pandemic preparedness. *Experimental & Molecular Medicine* 53(5):737–749.

Hatchett, R., M. Saville, M. Downham, T. Cueni, L. Bigger, P. Arthur, R. Suri, S. D. Prasad, and R. Bech Hansen. 2021. *Towards vaccinating the world: Landscape of current COVID-19 supply chain and manufacturing capacity, potential challenges, initial responses, and possible "solution space"—a discussion document.* https://www.ifpma.org/wp-content/uploads/2021/03/Summit_Landscape_Discussion_Document.pdf (accessed October 19, 2021).

Hay, A. J., and J. W. McCauley. 2018. The WHO Global Influenza Surveillance and Response System (GISRS)—a future perspective. *Influenza and Other Respiratory Viruses* 12(5):551–557.

Hendriks, J., M. Holleman, O. de Boer, P. de Jong, and W. Luytjes. 2011. An international technology platform for influenza vaccines. *Vaccine* 29:A8–A11.

HHS (U.S. Department of Health and Human Services). 2020a. *National Influenza Vaccine Modernization Strategy 2020–2030.* https://www.phe.gov/Preparedness/planning/nivms/Documents/nivms-2020-2030.pdf (accessed October 19, 2021).

HHS. 2020b. *Explaining Operation Warp Speed.* https://www.nihb.org/covid-19/wp-content/uploads/2020/08/Fact-sheet-operation-warp-speed.pdf (accessed October 19, 2021).

Honeycutt, A., T. Robinson, and C. Layton. 2005. *Influenza vaccine economics.* Triangle Park, NC: Research Triangle Institute.

Hotez, P. J., M. E. Bottazzi, and P. Yadav. 2021. Producing a vaccine requires more than a patent. *Foreign Affairs.* May 10.

Hoyt, K., and T. Johnston. 2021. *A plan to break the vaccine manufacturing bottleneck.* https://www.barrons.com/amp/articles/a-plan-to-break-the-vaccine-manufacturing-bottleneck-51621952245 (accessed October 19, 2021).

Hyder, A. A., M. A. Hyder, K. Nasir, and P. Ndebele. 2021. Inequitable COVID-19 vaccine distribution and its effects. *Bulletin of the World Health Organization* 99(6):406.

IRBM Group. 2020. *The Jenner Institute signs an agreement with Advent to develop a novel coronavirus vaccine.* https://www.irbm.com/news/the-jenner-institute-signs-an-agreement-with-advent-to-develop-a-novel-coronavirus-vaccine (accessed October 19, 2021).

Irwin, A. 2021. What it will take to vaccinate the world against COVID-19? *Nature* 592(7853):176–178.

Kis, Z., and Z. Rizvi. 2021. *How to make enough vaccine for the world in one year.* https://www.citizen.org/article/how-to-make-enough-vaccine-for-the-world-in-one-year (accessed October 19, 2021)

Knobler, S., C. Howell, M. Malchione, B. McCormick, and A. Mack. 2020. *Lessons from COVID-19: Advancing development of universal influenza vaccines.* Washington, DC: Sabin Vaccine Institute.

Krishtel, P., and R. Malpani. 2021. Suspend intellectual property rights for COVID-19 vaccines. *BMJ* 373:n1344.

Lemoine, C. H., R. V. Nidom, R. Ventura, S. Indrasari, I. Normalina, K. P. Santoso, F. Derouet, C. Barnier-Quer, G. Borchard, N. Collin, and C. A. Nidom. 2021. Better pandemic influenza preparedness through adjuvant technology transfer: Challenges and lessons learned. *Vaccines* 9(5):461.

Martin, C., and D. Lowery. 2020. mRNA vaccines: Intellectual property landscape. *Nature Reviews Drug Discoveries* 19(9):578.

Matthews, J. T. 2006. Egg-based production of influenza vaccine: 30 years of commercial experience. *The Bridge* 36(3).

Merck. 2021. *Merck to help produce Johnson & Johnson's COVID-19 vaccine; BARDA to provide Merck with funding to expand Merck's manufacturing capacity for COVID-19 vaccines and medicines.* Kenilworth, NJ: Merck. March 2.

Moderna. 2021. *Moderna provides business update and announces three new development programs in infectious disease vaccines.* https://investors.modernatx.com/news-releases/news-release-details/moderna-provides-business-update-and-announces-three-new (accessed October 19, 2021).

Murugan, S., S. Ponsekaran, L. Kannivel, L. N. Mangamoori, D. Chandran, S. Villuppanoor Alwar, C. Chakravarty, and S. K. Lal. 2013. Recombinant haemagglutinin protein of highly pathogenic avian influenza A(H5N1) virus expressed in *Pichia pastoris* elicits a neutralizing antibody response in mice. *Journal of Virological Methods* 187(1):20–25.

NASEM (National Academies of Sciences, Engineering, and Medicine). 2019. *Exploring lessons learned from a century of outbreaks: Readiness for 2030: Proceedings of a workshop.* Washington, DC: The National Academies Press.

Neal, J. C., K. Cappio, G. Woollett, R. Hughes IV, C. Chepigin, and Z. Klein. 2020. *Insights from the influenza vaccine market for COVID-19 vaccines.* https://avalere.com/insights/insights-from-the-influenza-vaccine-market-for-covid-19-vaccines (accessed October 19, 2021).

Ng, S. K. 2012. Current cell-based influenza vaccine production technology as pandemic contingency. *Human Vaccines & Immunotherapeutics* 8(2):267–271.

Novartis. 2021. *Novartis signs initial agreement to provide manufacturing capacity for Pfizer-BioNTech COVID-19 vaccine*. Basel, Switzerland: Novartis. January 29.

Our World in Data. 2021. *Coronavirus (COVID-19) vaccinations*. https://ourworldindata.org/covid-vaccinations#citation (accessed October 19, 2021).

Paden, C. R., Y. Tao, K. Queen, J. Zhang, Y. Li, A. Uehara, and S. Tong. 2020. Rapid, sensitive, full-genome sequencing of severe acute respiratory syndrome coronavirus 2. *Emerging Infectious Diseases* 26(10):2401–2405. https://doi.org/10.3201/eid2610.201800.

Palache, A., A. Abelin, R. Hollingsworth, W. Cracknell, C. Jacobs, T. Tsai, and P. Barbosa. 2017. Survey of distribution of seasonal influenza vaccine doses in 201 countries (2004–2015): The 2003 World Health Assembly resolution on seasonal influenza vaccination coverage and the 2009 influenza pandemic have had very little impact on improving influenza control and pandemic preparedness. *Vaccine* 35(36):4681–4686.

Palkonyay, L., and H. Fatima. 2016. A decade of adaptation: Regulatory contributions of the World Health Organization to the global action plan for influenza vaccines (2006–2016). *Vaccine* 34(45):5414–5419.

Paris, C. 2020. Supply-chain obstacles led to last month's cut to Pfizer's COVID-19 vaccine-rollout target. *The Wall Street Journal*. December 3.

PATH. 2019. *Supporting vaccine manufacturers to supply critical vaccines*. https://www.path.org/articles/supporting-vaccine-manufacturers-supply-critical-vaccines (accessed October 19, 2021).

Pfizer. 2020. *Pfizer and BioNTech to co-develop potential COVID-19 vaccine*. March 17. https://investors.pfizer.com/investor-news/press-release-details/2020/Pfizer-and-BioNTech-to-Co-Develop-Potential-COVID-19-Vaccine/default.aspx (accessed October 19, 2021).

Pfizer. 2021. *New RNA technology could get the flu vaccine right, every year*. https://www.pfizer.com/news/featured_stories/featured_stories_detail/new_rna_technology_could_get_the_flu_vaccine_right_every_year (accessed October 19, 2021).

Plotkin, S., J. M. Robinson, G. Cunningham, R. Iqbal, and S. Larsen. 2017. The complexity and cost of vaccine manufacturing - an overview. *Vaccine* 35(33):4064–4071.

Rajaram, S., C. Boikos, D. K. Gelone, and A. Gandhi. 2020. Influenza vaccines: The potential benefits of cell-culture isolation and manufacturing. *Therapeutic Advances in Vaccines and Immunotherapy* 8:2515135520908121.

Rappuoli, R., E. De Gregorio, G. Del Giudice, S. Phogat, S. Pecetta, M. Pizza, and E. Hanon. 2021. Vaccinology in the post–COVID-19 era. *Proceedings of the National Academy of Sciences* 118(3):e2020368118.

Rele, S. 2021. COVID-19 vaccine development during pandemic: Gap analysis, opportunities, and impact on future emerging infectious disease development strategies. *Human Vaccines & Immunotherapeutics* 17(4):1122–1127.

Rockman, S., K. Laurie, and I. Barr. 2020. Pandemic influenza vaccines: What did we learn from the 2009 pandemic and are we better prepared now? *Vaccines* 8(2):211.

Rosa, S. S., D. M. F. Prazeres, A. M. Azevedo, and M. P. C. Marques. 2021. mRNA vaccines manufacturing: Challenges and bottlenecks. *Vaccine* 39(16):2190–2200.

Saelens, X., P. Vanlandschoot, W. Martinet, M. Maras, S. Neirynck, R. Contreras, W. Fiers, and W. M. Jou. 1999. Protection of mice against a lethal influenza virus challenge after immunization with yeast-derived secreted influenza virus hemagglutinin. *European Journal of Biochemistry* 260(1):166–175.

Sanofi. 2021. *Sanofi to provide support to BioNTech in manufacturing their COVID-19 vaccine to help address public health needs*. Paris, France: Sanofi. January 27.

Schmidt, C. 2021. New COVID vaccines need absurd amounts of material and labor. *Scientific American*. January 4.

Shang, Y., H. Li, and R. Zhang. 2021. Effects of pandemic outbreak on economies: Evidence from business history context. *Frontiers in Public Health* 9(146).

Soema, P. C., R. Kompier, J.-P. Amorij, and G. F. A. Kersten. 2015. Current and next generation influenza vaccines: Formulation and production strategies. *European Journal of Pharmaceutics and Biopharmaceutics* 94:251–263.

Sparrow, E., J. G. Wood, C. Chadwick, A. T. Newall, S. Torvaldsen, A. Moen, and G. Torelli. 2021. Global production capacity of seasonal and pandemic influenza vaccines in 2019. *Vaccine* 39(3):512–520.

Tenforde, M. W., S. M. Olson, W. H. Self, H. K. Talbot, C. J. Lindsell, J. S. Steingrub, N. I. Shapiro, A. A. Ginde, D. J. Douin, M. E. Prekker, S. M. Brown, I. D. Peltan, M. N. Gong, A. Mohamed, A. Khan, M. C. Exline, D. C. Files, K. W. Gibbs, W. B. Stubblefield, J. D. Casey, T. W. Rice, C. G. Grijalva, D. N. Hager, A. Shehu, N. Qadir, S. Y. Chang, J. G. Wilson, M. Gaglani, K. Murthy, N. Calhoun, A. S. Monto, E. T. Martin, A. Malani, R. K. Zimmerman, F. P. Silveira, D. B. Middleton, Y. Zhu, D. Wyatt, M. Stephenson, A. Baughman, K. N. Womack, K. W. Hart, M. Kobayashi, J. R. Verani, and M. M. Patel. 2021. Effectiveness of Pfizer-BioNTech and Moderna vaccines against COVID-19 among hospitalized adults aged ≥65 years—United States, January–March 2021. *Morbidity and Mortality Weekly Report* 70(18):674–679.

WHO (World Health Organization). 2019. *Global influenza strategy 2019–2030*. Geneva, Switzerland: World Health Organization.

WHO. 2021a. *Establishment of a COVID-19 mRNA vaccine technology transfer hub to scale up global manufacturing*. https://www.who.int/news-room/articles-detail/establishment-of-a-covid-19-mrna vaccine-technology-transfer-hub-to-scale-up-global-manufacturing (accessed October 19, 2021).

WHO. 2021b. *The effects of virus variants on COVID-19 vaccines*. https://www.who.int/news-room/feature-stories/detail/the-effects-of-virus-variants-on-covid-19-vaccines (accessed October 19, 2021).

Williams, S. R., A. J. Driscoll, H. M. LeBuhn, W. H. Chen, K. M. Neuzil, and J. R. Ortiz. 2021. National routine adult immunisation programmes among World Health Organization member states: An assessment of health systems to deploy COVID-19 vaccines. *Eurosurveillance* 26(17):2001195.

Woolston, C. 2021. "Does anyone have any of these?": Lab-supply shortages strike amid global pandemic. *Nature*. https://pubmed.ncbi.nlm.nih.gov/33750928 (accessed October 19, 2021).

5

Regulatory Science

An effective regulatory process, built on strong regulatory science, is essential to the development and deployment of safe and effective vaccines. It is also necessary for public trust in vaccination.

This chapter addresses the fourth of the four dimensions of vaccine research, development, and manufacturing examined by the committee. It begins by describing the role of regulatory science in the development of COVID-19 vaccines. The chapter then considers how lessons learned from the development of COVID-19 vaccines (shown in Box 5-1) can be applied to both seasonal and pandemic influenza vaccines in the dimension of regulatory science. The final section presents recommendations drawn from these findings.

BOX 5-1
Regulatory Science: Lessons Learned from the COVID-19 Pandemic

- Clear guidance was provided to manufacturers on the minimum efficacy levels that vaccine candidates would need to meet for emergency approval.
- Harmonization of labeling requirements such as QR codes and fill dates bolstered global coordination and regulatory oversight.
- People known to be pregnant and children younger than 16 years were excluded from phase III trials, leading to gaps in knowledge and public health recommendations.

continued

BOX 5-1 Continued

- Companies and regulators identified ways to conduct chemistry, manufacturing, and controls virtually, to ensure rigorous safety standards were being met.
- Political interference and other external factors affected public perception of vaccines and created significant vaccine hesitancy.
- Communication challenges between manufacturers, regulatory bodies, and the public when reporting on adverse reactions undermined public confidence in the vaccines.
- Regulators allowed for a rolling review of data during the developmental stages of the vaccines to accelerate emergency use and conditional marketing authorization procedures.
- The use of a single safety monitoring board provided harmonization and coordinated oversight during clinical trials.

REGULATORY SCIENCE AND THE DEVELOPMENT OF COVID-19 VACCINES

When SARS-CoV-2 was identified in early 2020, regulators around the world had only modest prior experience with coronavirus vaccines. Not only were there no approved vaccines for this family of viruses, but there were also no established correlates of protection and only minimal experience related to safety. To address these challenges, the U.S. Food and Drug Administration (FDA), the World Health Organization (WHO), and other leading agencies quickly established a process that supported the development of multiple safe and effective vaccines on innovative platforms at unprecedented speed. Key regulatory issues have included guidance for manufacturing, preclinical data, and clinical trials on the pathway to Emergency Use Authorization and licensure; coordination with regulated industry; public communications and transparency; and global collaboration and coordination, particularly with respect to emerging safety issues. Lessons from each of these areas are relevant to the challenge of developing safe and effective vaccines for pandemic influenza.

It should be noted that the starting point for regulators for the development of pandemic influenza vaccines is quite different from the starting point for COVID-19 vaccines. There are already multiple licensed influenza vaccines, established correlates of immunity, and the opportunity to test new seasonal influenza vaccine platforms through phase III trials every year. At the same time, current vaccines and vaccine platforms are insufficient to meet the global need for pandemic influenza, which therefore is the focus of this chapter.

Regulatory Guidance

Soon after the discovery of SARS-CoV-2, as scientists around the world began the research into candidate vaccines, regulators started to plan the regulatory pathway from preclinical data to large trials to establish safety and efficacy. In June 2020, FDA released guidance covering necessary chemistry, manufacturing and controls for vaccine production, nonclinical studies relevant to novel platforms including mRNA, and clinical trials (FDA, 2020). Among the topics covered were how vaccine manufacturers could assess the potential for vaccine-associated enhanced respiratory disease, an early concern of some coronavirus experts.

This document established rigorous standards for phase III clinical trials. It required that vaccines reduce COVID-19 by at least 50 percent, with 95 percent confidence intervals demonstrating at least a 30 percent reduction; as a result, phase III clinical trials had to involve tens of thousands of patients. FDA also required that the studies include a diversity of patients, including large numbers of older adults most at risk of death from COVID-19.

A subsequent FDA guidance, first issued in October 2020, set standards for the Emergency Use Authorization of COVID-19 vaccines. This guidance required substantial evidence of clinical efficacy, consistent with the earlier communication, and added a requirement of at least 2 months of median follow-up time for safety assessment (FDA, 2021). FDA released this guidance after an extraordinary public dispute with the White House, which involved the president of the United States accusing the agency of setting excessively high standards in order to hurt him politically (LaFraniere and Weiland, 2020). Seven former FDA commissioners wrote to defend the agency against such political interference (Califf et al., 2020).

Regulators in other nations overseeing the development of vaccines, including Russia and China, did not publicly release their standards for vaccine development. The Medicines and Healthcare Products Regulatory Agency in the United Kingdom did not require clinical trials to be as large as those for FDA review; however, the small number of older adults in initial trials for AstraZeneca vaccines later led to confusion about whether the vaccine worked in older adults and affected initial country decisions on adoption (Davis, 2021).

The initial U.S. standards had some noticeable gaps. FDA did not require early study of the vaccines in children or people known to be pregnant, which led to gaps in knowledge and public health recommendations in the United States that people who are pregnant make their own decisions with limited evidence (Klein et al., 2021; Mandavilli and Rabin, 2021). Standard setting is a dynamic process, responding to emerging evidence of safety, efficacy, and immunogenicity. At the time of this report's publication, for example, the standards for pediatric vaccine development remain in flux, as scientists work to establish the appropriate dose, given the robust immune response to SARS-CoV-2 among children (Johnson, 2021).

Coordination with Regulated Industry

With a novel, deadly virus moving across the planet, regulators altered their usual approach from requiring a single submission to allowing sequential submission and review of information from vaccine developers. Agencies conducted rolling reviews during clinical development, with nearly continuous exchange of data between industry and national regulators (CDC, 2021a). The need for such coordination was heightened by the threat of the pandemic itself. Chemistry, manufacturing, and control (CMC) processes are ideally performed at the manufacturing location. However, this was not always possible because of nationwide stay-at-home orders and mandates to limit face-to-face interaction. During the COVID-19 pandemic, companies and regulators identified ways to conduct the oversight of the CMC online, with regulators inspecting manufacturing facilities at times via video call (Stewart et al., 2021).

Coordination extended to key public statements. In September 2020, for example, nine leading vaccine companies pledged to support high safety standards and to not file for regulatory authorization or approval until established clinical benchmarks had been met (Loftus and Hopkins, 2020).

Public Communications and Transparency

It is not enough to know a vaccine is safe and effective. The public must trust in the process of vaccine development and appreciate the evidence that supports recommendations for use. This distinction reflects the public health wisdom that "vaccines don't save lives, vaccination saves lives."

Several communications challenges occurred during the clinical development of SARS-CoV-2 vaccines. In September 2020, U.S. and UK regulators put clinical trials for the AstraZeneca vaccine on hold because of a suspected serious adverse reaction. Information emerged about the situation from the company's chief executive officer, through his private briefings with investors (Feurstein, 2020). However, regulators provided few details, even as the trials were restarted. Meanwhile, newspaper accounts documented behind-the-scenes disputes between company and government officials (Robbins and Mueller, 2020).

Communications issues intensified around the release of trial results, as companies issued press releases limited to topline data, and politicians extolled the virtues of their own country's vaccines and debated who won the "vaccine race." Public confidence may have been undermined by the perception that political one-upmanship had influenced regulatory decision making.

Transparency supports the credibility of regulatory agencies (Sharfstein, 2020). At the country level, regulators differed in what they revealed publicly about the regulatory process. In the United States, prior to making decisions on Emergency Use Authorization, FDA released its own analyses of company data and convened public meetings of its independent advisory committee. These meetings included presentations from regulatory scientists and company officials, with extensive questions from the committee members and an opportunity for public comment. This process led to robust news coverage of the strong independent endorsements of the vaccines' safety and efficacy (Sharfstein et al., 2021). China and Russia, by contrast, initially provided little explanation or data to support the use of their vaccines, which has contributed to confusion about these vaccines within and outside of these countries (Cohen and Moutinho, 2021; Sharfstein et al., 2021).

Other transparency issues related to the disclosure of study protocols are the release of clinical trial data and the regulatory pathway to licensure. Under public pressure, several manufacturers released the protocols for their phase III clinical trials, which boosted confidence in their rigorous approach (COVID vaccine confidence requires radical transparency, 2020). Not all manufacturers have committed to making clinical trial data available to independent researchers. In the United States, obscure reasoning behind the delay in licensing vaccines has led to calls for more clarity on timing standards for licensure (Topol, 2021).

Global Collaboration and Coordination

The rapid pace of COVID-19 vaccine development has stressed the global regulatory system. A limited number of experienced and well-resourced regulatory agencies have led in the regulatory review of COVID-19 vaccines, with many other national authorities relying on these assessments and the work of WHO. Over the course of the pandemic, the need for greater global collaboration and coordination has become clear. Opportunities exist for greater regulatory harmonization, improved sharing of data on manufacturing concerns, and a more coordinated response to emerging safety issues. It is challenging for regulatory agencies to scale-up for a pandemic response and then reduce or redistribute resource expenditures after the pandemic response. Addressing this challenge could help in future pandemic responses.

During the pandemic, the COVAX effort played an important role in promoting global coordination in regulatory oversight. COVAX supported harmonization of certain documents and processes, such as vaccine label requirements for QR codes and fill dates. COVAX also required that vaccines for distribution qualify for an emergency use listing by WHO. Steps to an emergency use listing include an independent assessment of clinical trial data by the technical advisory group comprised of regulatory experts from around the world. Moreover, according to WHO, "as part of the Emergency Use Listing process, the company producing the vaccine must commit to continue to generate data to enable full licensure and WHO prequalification of the vaccine" (WHO, 2021). However, COVAX was limited in its ability to harmonize requirements across leading national regulatory agencies. At the same time, some vaccines were not able to be listed by WHO because of inadequate local standards, and production problems created international shortages. A surge in COVID-19 cases in India disrupted an anticipated global supply, and after a U.S. production plant experienced a variety of production problems, including cross contamination with another vaccine, global distribution of millions of doses came to a halt (Swaine and Rowland, 2021).

The challenge of global regulatory coordination during COVID-19 may be best illustrated by the variety of regulatory response to emerging safety issues. In early 2021, it became clear that two adenovirus-vectored vaccines produced by AstraZeneca and Johnson & Johnson were associated with a rare but severe syndrome of thrombosis with thrombocytopenia (Long et al., 2021; Tsilingiris et al., 2021). In response, some nations suspended use of these vaccines altogether, others limited the vaccines to older adults, and still others added warnings to the vaccine labels (Fox, 2021; Weiland et al., 2021). The European Medicines Agency had recommended continuing the use of the vaccine, and the European Union asked its members to "speak with one voice" on the topic. Nonetheless, every country in the European Union made its own considerations and recommendations for the use of this vaccine (Euronews, 2021). This varied response, and the resulting absence of a cohesive unified public message, may have undermined vaccine confidence.

REGULATORY SCIENCE: APPLYING LESSONS FROM THE DEVELOPMENT OF COVID-19 VACCINES TO VACCINES FOR INFLUENZA

The rapid development of COVID-19 vaccines on novel platforms has important implications for the development of new vaccines against pandemic influenza. For example, the tremendous success of mRNA vaccines has created hope that similar success and scale can be achieved for influenza (Anand and Stahel, 2021). However, limited data are available for mRNA influenza vaccines, and both safety and efficacy will have to be demonstrated for these platforms (Bever, 2021). Success will require regulators to rethink established practices and expectations for influenza vaccines to support rapid innovation. Just as the time is now to support urgent basic research for vaccines for pandemic influenza, work on a companion regulatory process cannot be delayed. This section considers the application of lessons learned from regulatory experience in the four areas discussed above for COVID-19 vaccines: regulatory guidance, coordination with regulated industry, public communications and transparency, and global collaboration and coordination.

Regulatory Guidance and Coordination with Regulated Industry

The example of COVID-19 demonstrates how regulators can work with the scientific community and the pharmaceutical industry to establish guidance for the development of novel vaccine platforms (including novel adjuvants) for influenza. A logical starting point for this guidance is a pathway for seasonal influenza vaccines, from preclinical studies through licensure, informed by the best practices during COVID-19 of rapid data sharing and review. In formulating this guidance, a key consideration is that the existing hemagglutination inhibition (HI) assay may be potentially insufficient or possibly not relevant to new platforms, and as a result, it may be necessary to conduct clinical trials to generate data related to other potential correlates of protection (van Els et al., 2014). The existence of an accelerated pathway to licensure based on HI can, nevertheless, facilitate development of novel influenza vaccines so this existing pathway must remain in place, to which new pathways can be added.

Turning to the rapid adaptation of seasonal influenza vaccines for pandemic influenza, regulators will want to consider what data can be acquired in the interpandemic period, such as phase I and phase II data for vaccines targeting common pandemic subtypes (Krammer and Palese, 2014). Important as well will be laying out an approach to confirming safety and efficacy as quickly as possible following the recognition of an influenza pandemic. This guidance will need to be dynamic and evolving based on what is learned through the development of these platforms for seasonal influenza.

Conclusion 5-1: An important role for regulators is to formulate and/or update guidance for the development of both seasonal and pandemic influenza vaccines to provide more clarity on expectations for postauthorization/postapproval confirmatory efficacy studies. Ideally, a successful demonstration of safety and effectiveness for seasonal influenza vaccines, combined with the establishment of new correlates of protection, will inform a development pathway for pandemic vaccines that can be accomplished in a matter of months during a pandemic without requiring full phase III clinical trials. In this case, the guidance will need to establish expectations for postauthorization confirmation of efficacy.

Guidance from regulators will also need to incorporate standards for the inclusion of diverse populations, including pregnant individuals and children, in clinical trials (see Chapter 3). Influenza is known to be a serious threat to people who are pregnant and children, so it is essential that these groups be included early on in clinical trials for influenza vaccines (CDC, 2021b; Poehling et al., 2013). For pandemic vaccine development, guidance can be contingent upon the risk of the infectious agent to each population to stratify the most affected populations for early investigations. Close monitoring of early studies should balance the need for including key populations with the urgency of pandemic response.

Conclusion 5-2: Guidance from regulators can help advance the inclusion in clinical trials of diverse population groups, especially those for whom influenza poses a significant risk, such as children and people who are pregnant.

Public Communications and Transparency

Applying the lessons from COVID-19 vaccine development, regulatory agencies, and WHO can commit to transparency as a key principle in oversight of influenza vaccines. Regulators can provide updates on the status of clinical trials (including basic information about clinical holds), release their own analyses of company data, provide for independent and public review of the data by advisory committees, and offer opportunities for questions and answers from the public and the news media.

For their part, vaccine manufacturers can release the protocols of pivotal clinical trials and make trial data available to qualified researchers, such as through the Yale Open Data Access project (YODA, 2021). The industry can also adopt a code of conduct for announcements of study results that emphasizes the preliminary nature of the findings and the role of independent review by regulators. It will also be important for such a code to support the ability of regulators to rapidly correct misstatements by commercial interests.

Conclusion 5-3: Careful conduct of public communications and transparency can help the public understand the development process for influenza vaccines and counter any misinformation to which they may be exposed.

Global Collaborations and Coordination

Just as for COVID-19 vaccines, international collaboration in regulatory science is essential for the development and safe implementation of vaccines for pandemic influenza. To this end, COVAX and WHO can continue and expand their roles for pandemic influenza, supporting harmonization where possible for vaccine manufacturers. WHO can act as a coordinator of critical areas of data sharing between regulators, including the sharing of data on efficacy and safety, postmarketing surveillance data, and information on product quality. WHO can coordinate with international regulatory agencies to develop core global regulatory standards for Emergency Use Authorization to provide a strong, stable, global vaccine supply in a pandemic. Such broad promulgation of basic standards for production can reduce the chance that vaccines will not receive authorization or will experience serious manufacturing quality problems.

Conclusion 5-4: There is a strong need to develop a robust and coordinated review process for influenza vaccines with consistent standards globally to minimize vaccine development delays and mitigate the credibility issues arising from variable decisions across countries.

National regulatory agencies value their ability to make their own authorization and licensing decisions and fashion their own responses to emerging safety issues and are unlikely to relinquish it. Indeed, risk–benefit analyses for the use of vaccines include multiple country-level factors that affect the results. For example, the prevalence of the virus in a specific region and the availability of other vaccines with a potential different safety and efficacy profile are variables that may lead to a difference in risk–benefit outcomes across countries and regions.

At the same time, when national regulatory agencies make different decisions about the same vaccines, confusion and vaccine hesitancy can result (Petersen, 2021). The committee therefore emphasizes the importance of coordination among regulators in explaining their decisions to the public. Transparency, as discussed above, is an essential element of this coordination. In addition, when explaining the decisions made for their own countries, regulators can acknowledge that circumstances may be different in other countries. Wherever possible, establishing a communication plan will help the public understand different recommendations on the same vaccines in different countries.

Conclusion 5-5: Risk–benefit analyses and regulatory decisions regarding influenza vaccines can be expected to differ across countries and regions. Explaining such differences to the public is an important part of the communications and transparency discussed above.

RECOMMENDATIONS

Recommendation 5-1: The U.S. Food and Drug Administration and other national regulators (e.g., European Medicines Agency) working with the scientific community and pharmaceutical industry should enhance comprehensive guidance for the development of influenza vaccines on novel platforms through Emergency Use Authorization to full licensure. This guidance should provide pathways for seasonal and pandemic influenza.

Recommendation 5-2: The U.S. Food and Drug Administration and other national regulators (e.g., European Medicines Agency) should commit to transparency in the oversight of clinical trials, review of data, authorization, and approval of pandemic influenza vaccines, including the release of facility inspection findings, clinical trial protocols, and clinical data that are the basis of decision making. Regulators should convene independent advisory committees to systematically review data, make recommendations, and build public understanding and confidence prior to the authorization or approval of novel vaccines.

Recommendation 5-3: The World Health Organization and the International Coalition of Medicines Regulatory Authorities should encourage and support the coordination between regulatory and public health agencies (e.g., the U.S. Centers for Disease Control and Prevention, the European Centre for Disease Prevention and Control, the China Center for Disease Control and Prevention, and the Africa Centres for Disease Control and Prevention) when announcing different decisions on the same or similar vaccines, to explain the different underlying circumstances and judgments.

Recommendation 5-4: Vaccine manufacturers should adopt a code of conduct for press releases and other communications regarding vaccine trial results and other matters that emphasizes the critical role of regulatory review

REFERENCES

Anand, P., and V. P. Stahel. 2021. The safety of COVID-19 mRNA vaccines: A review. *Patient Safety in Surgery* 15(1):20.

Bever, L. 2021. Coronavirus vaccine technology is paving the way for a whole new approach to flu shots. *The Washington Post*. April 11.

Califf, R., S. Gottlieb, M. Hamburg, J. Henney, D. Kessler, M. McClellan, and A. von Eschenbach. 2020. 7 former FDA commissioners: The Trump administration is undermining the credibility of the FDA. *The Washington Post*. September 29.

CDC (Centers for Disease Control and Prevention). 2021a. *Developing COVID-19 vaccines*. https://www.cdc.gov/coronavirus/2019-ncov/vaccines/distributing/steps-ensure-safety.html (accessed October 19, 2021).

CDC. 2021b. *Flu & pregnancy*. https://www.cdc.gov/flu/highrisk/pregnant.htm (accessed October 19, 2021).

Cohen, J., and S. Moutinho. 2021. Third time's the charm? Brazil scales back efficacy claims for COVID-19 vaccine from China. *Science*. https://www.science.org/content/article/third-time-s-charm-brazil-scales-back-efficacy-claims-covid-19-vaccine-china (accessed October 20, 2021).

COVID vaccine confidence requires radical transparency. 2020. *Nature* 586(7827):8.

Davis, N. 2021. Why has Germany advised against Oxford/AstraZeneca jab for over-65s? *The Guardian*. January 28.

Euronews. 2021. *Countries change tack on AstraZeneca vaccine despite EU call for unity*. https://www.euronews.com/2021/04/07/countries-change-tack-on-astrazeneca-vaccine-despite-eu-call-for-unity (accessed October 19, 2021).

FDA (U.S. Food and Drug Administration). 2020. *Development and licensure of vaccines to prevent COVID-19*. https://www.fda.gov/regulatory-information/search-fda-guidance-documents/development-and-licensure-vaccines-prevent-covid-19 (accessed October 19, 2021).

FDA. 2021. *Emergency Use Authorization for vaccines to prevent COVID-19*. https://www.fda.gov/regulatory-information/search-fda-guidance-documents/emergency-use-authorization-vaccines-prevent-covid-19 (accessed October 19, 2021).

Feurstein, A. 2020. *COVID-19 vaccine trial participant had serious neurological symptoms, but could be discharged today, AstraZeneca CEO says*. https://www.statnews.com/2020/09/09/astrazeneca-covid19-vaccine-trial-hold-patient-report (accessed October 19, 2021).

Fox, M. 2021. *CDC, FDA lift pause on using J&J's coronavirus vaccine, add safety warning*. https://www.cnn.com/2021/04/23/health/johnson-vaccine-acip-recommendation/index.html (accessed October 19, 2021).

Johnson, C. Y. 2021. FDA advisers debate standards on a coronavirus vaccine for young children. *The Washington Post*. June 10.

Klein, S. L., P. S. Creisher, and I. Burd. 2021. COVID-19 vaccine testing in pregnant females is necessary. *Journal of Clinical Investigation* 131(5).

Krammer, F., and P. Palese. 2014. Universal influenza virus vaccines: Need for clinical trials. *Nature Immunology* 15(1):3–5.

LaFraniere, S., and N. Weiland. 2020. White House blocks new coronavirus vaccine guidelines. *The New York Times*. October 23.

Loftus, P., and J. S. Hopkins. 2020. COVID-19 vaccine developers prepare joint pledge on safety, standards. *The Wall Street Journal*. September 4.

Long, B., R. Bridwell, and M. Gottlieb. 2021. Thrombosis with thrombocytopenia syndrome associated with COVID-19 vaccines. *American Journal of Emergency Medicine* 49:58–61.

Mandavilli, A., and R. C. Rabin. 2021. Pregnant women get conflicting advice on COVID-19 vaccines. *The New York Times*. January 28.

Petersen, M., F. J. Jørgensen, A. Bor, and M. F. Lindholt. 2021. *Did the suspension of the AstraZeneca-vaccine decrease vaccine acceptance?* Aarhus, Denmark: Aarhus University.

Poehling, K. A., K. M. Edwards, M. R. Griffin, P. G. Szilagyi, M. A. Staat, M. K. Iwane, B. M. Snively, C. K. Suerken, C. B. Hall, G. A. Weinberg, S. S. Chaves, Y. Zhu, M. M. McNeal, and C. B. Bridges. 2013. The burden of influenza in young children, 2004–2009. *Pediatrics* 131(2):207–216.

Robbins, R., and B. Mueller. 2020. After admitting mistake, AstraZeneca faces difficult questions about its vaccine. *The New York Times.* November 26.

Sharfstein, J. 2020. How the FDA should protect its integrity from politics. *Nature* 585(7824):161.

Sharfstein, J. M., J. L. Goodman, and L. Borio. 2021. The US regulatory system and COVID-19 vaccines: The importance of a strong and capable FDA. *JAMA* 325(12):1153–1154.

Stewart, J., P. Honig, L. AlJuburi, D. Autor, S. Berger, P. Brady, H. Fitton, C. Garner, M. Garvin, M. Hukkelhoven, R. Kowalski, S. Milligan, L. O'Dowd, E. Reilly, K. Roberts, A. S. Robertson, M. Taisey, R. Thakkar, K. Van Baelen, and M. Wegner. 2021. COVID-19: A catalyst to accelerate global regulatory transformation. *Clinical Pharmacology and Therapeutics* 109(6):1390–1392.

Swaine, J., and C. Rowland. 2021. Emergent plant that ruined Johnson & Johnson vaccine doses had prior FDA violations. *The Washington Post.* April 1.

Topol, E. J. 2021. It's time for the FDA to fully approve the mRNA vaccines. *The New York Times.* July 1.

Tsilingiris, D., N. G. Vallianou, I. Karampela, and M. Dalamaga. 2021. Vaccine induced thrombotic thrombocytopenia: The shady chapter of a success story. *Metabolism Open* 11:100101.

van Els, C., S. Mjaaland, L. Næss, J. Sarkadi, E. Gonczol, K. S. Korsholm, J. Hansen, J. de Jonge, G. Kersten, J. Warner, A. Semper, C. Kruiswijk, and F. Oftung. 2014. Fast vaccine design and development based on correlates of protection (COPs). *Human Vaccines & Immunotherapeutics* 10(7):1935–1948.

Weiland, N., S. LaFraniere, and C. Zimmer. 2021. Johnson & Johnson vaccinations paused after rare clotting cases emerge. *The New York Times.* April 14.

WHO (World Health Organization). 2021. *WHO lists additional COVID-19 vaccine for emergency use and issues interim policy recommendations.* May 7, 2021. https://www.who.int/news/item/07-05-2021-who-lists-additional-covid-19-vaccine-for-emergency-use-and-issues-interim-policy-recommendations (accessed October 20, 2021).

YODA (Yale Open Data Access) Project. 2021. *Welcome to the YODA project.* https://yoda.yale.edu (accessed October 19, 2021).

6

A Blueprint for Action

Given the many years of research and the well-oiled machine for vaccine production, the world is better prepared for the next impending influenza outbreak than it was for the COVID-19 pandemic. Nonetheless, lessons learned from the response to COVID-19 can help ensure preparedness for a future influenza pandemic. Vaccine research and development (R&D) took major steps forward in 2020 and 2021, with novel vaccine platforms obtaining Emergency Use Authorization that enabled the rapid immunization of millions of people to curb the COVID-19 pandemic. Yet, while vaccines were available for COVID-19 within 1 year of its onset, there remains significant room for improvements that would speed up vaccine research, development, and manufacturing. Having vaccines earlier in a future influenza pandemic could significantly reduce both the burden of disease and the social and economic consequences. Valuable resources have been developed, such as the Influenza Vaccines Roadmap, developed by the Center for Infectious Disease Research and Policy, to develop a framework for expedient R&D of influenza vaccines (CIDRAP, 2021). This report builds on existing work and investigates what lessons can be learned from the development of COVID-19 vaccines given the current state of influenza vaccine research.

During its deliberations, the committee explored a range of topics that it decided to categorize in the dimensions of basic and translational science, clinical science, manufacturing science, and regulatory science. The recommendations presented in this chapter can serve collectively as a blueprint for action to accelerate the vaccine development process, increase access to vaccines, and limit global vaccine inequity. These recommendations are designed to respond to the priority needs for seasonal and pandemic influenza identified below.

PRIORITY NEEDS FOR ADVANCING THE DEVELOPMENT OF VACCINES FOR SEASONAL AND PANDEMIC INFLUENZA

Investments to Support Influenza Vaccine Research and Development

Continuous funding streams are essential for vaccine R&D. During pandemics, funding is generally sufficient, but it often decreases considerably once a pandemic has ended, resulting in halted or limited research. Seasonal influenza vaccines have low to moderate effectiveness and require renewal every year because of antigenic drift of the virus and the short-lived immunity induced by vaccines (Gerdil, 2003; Rajaram et al., 2020). Today, influenza vaccines are based largely on inactivated virus grown in embryonated chicken eggs (Bender, 2019; Gerdil, 2003). Even though this is a successful way of producing vaccines, more effective vaccines are urgently needed, as are novel vaccine platforms for quick access during a pandemic.

A priority need, then, is for the allocation of a continuous and permanent stream of funding to support the development of broadly protective influenza vaccines, as well as novel vaccine platform technologies. For pandemic preparedness, the additional development of vaccines targeting conserved epitopes, or other types of broadly protective vaccine constructs, such as supraseasonal, pan-subtype, or pan-group, is vital to developing a pandemic-ready stockpile. Given the great potential of the mRNA vaccine platform, as illustrated by its use to produce two successful vaccines for COVID-19 within 12 months, further study of this platform for production of influenza vaccines is clearly warranted. Additionally, recombinant protein vaccines are of interest for influenza, and so it would be valuable to invest in improving the responsiveness of this platform. Adjuvants are another valuable area of investment because of their effects on antigen sparing for egg-based, cell-based, and recombinant vaccines. Efficacy data from animal models and early clinical trials are required to establish the most suitable platforms for investments.

Considerations in determining the best platforms for further development include issues associated with expansion of manufacturing capacity and feasibility of scale-up in low- and middle-income countries (LMICs), as well as effectiveness, speed, and cost. For each new platform, standardized assays, reagents, and animal models will be needed. Research on surrogate markers of protection for each platform would facilitate the establishment of the regulatory requirements for such vaccines.

Beyond the development of novel platforms and next-generation vaccines, significant investment in research aimed at identifying methods for overcoming viral drift effects and optimizing adjuvant manufacturing could yield knowledge that would aid in the rational design of vaccines and, more specifically, the development of vaccines for particular subpopulations.

Finally, building a framework for collaboration or using an existing organization to distribute know-how domestically and internationally would provide vital support for global vaccine development.

Clinical Research into Novel Influenza Vaccines to Increase Pandemic Preparedness

The main gap in the development of next-generation influenza vaccines is the clinical development. Given the costly nature of such studies and the current approval process for seasonal influenza vaccines, there is little incentive for the industry to conduct such trials. Seasonal egg-based vaccines need to be complemented by candidate vaccine and vaccine adjuvant combinations that have undergone multicenter international trials to establish safety and immunogenicity. The conduct of clinical trials throughout the world, from the early stages of development, would fill the clinical funding gap and ensure global preparedness.

To this end, public-sector investments are essential to improve the data-sharing infrastructure so vaccine manufacturing centers could mobilize quickly and efficiently (such as using the highly effective nongovernmental GISAID data-sharing structure), which in turn would help shorten the time from sequence discovery and publication to global distribution of vaccines. Financial aid could stimulate vaccine manufacturers to take a risk-based approach to pandemic influenza preparedness, understanding that the investments made would be a form of insurance that would limit the costs of the next impending influenza outbreak. To qualify for these funding initiatives, manufacturers would be required to participate in R&D, data sharing, technology adaptation, and training activities with international partners. In addition, it would be important to stimulate technology transfer for both scale-up and scale-out. Scientific evidence supporting design strategies such as WHO prequalification or licensing could be used to reduce risk.

Many countries, in particular LMICs, do not have seasonal influenza vaccine programs as there is a low perceived urgency of the threat of influenza relative to the cost (Ortiz and Neuzil, 2019; Williams et al., 2021). Figures 4-2 and 4-3 show the prevalence of adult immunization programs in the world and reflect that many countries have influenza programs in place, particularly in Europe and the Americas. However, there appears to be a significant disparity in the existence of these programs between high-income countries (HICs) and LMICs. However, the costs and impact of seasonal influenza are high, and the expansion of seasonal programs would improve pandemic preparedness. Therefore, burden-of-disease studies, including cost–benefit analyses and analyses of economic productivity losses, are needed to create a case for local governments to adopt a seasonal vaccine program.

For clinical studies of novel seasonal influenza vaccines, accurate determination of postapproval vaccine effectiveness will be essential. Furthermore, postapproval safety monitoring will need to be performed on a global scale to detect any safety signals. Important priorities include sustaining local networks of clinical trials and research capacities, increasing the involvement of LMICs in clinical trials, and helping LMICs develop distribution capacities. A global coordinated pharmacovigilance system is needed to complement this work, with an increase in surveillance and pharmacovigilance systems in LMICs, providing the ability to calculate background rates, conduct rapid case-control studies, and assess subpopulations.

To enable clinical trials in LMICs, a wide variety of stakeholders will have to collaborate in a global network of funding and coordination to ensure that challenges are overcome and duplication of effort is minimized. Given the potential for competing research priorities among stakeholders, regional and international research groups, nongovernmental organizations, humanitarian organizations, international agencies such as WHO, and funding agencies, coordination will be key in moving the field forward.

Expanding Influenza Vaccine Manufacturing Capacity

The great majority of the world's vaccine manufacturing capacity is based in HICs (Sparrow et al., 2021). Even though there are some big players in LMICs, it is essential to expand manufacturing capacity in these regions. The COVID-19 pandemic has shown that countries and regions with manufacturing capacity have an advantage in early access to pandemic vaccines, and during the COVID-19 pandemic, vaccine nationalism delayed the equitable global distribution of vaccines (Hyder et al., 2021). International action is required to build on the momentum of and attention to COVID-19 vaccine development to strengthen the manufacturing landscape for influenza vaccines.

Organizations and governments can help meet this need by supporting and encouraging vaccine manufacturers to prioritize and harmonize influenza vaccine development and manufacturing capacity. The approach taken by the Coalition for Epidemic Preparedness Innovations (CEPI) to address the COVID-19 pandemic provides a valuable model for effectively mobilizing and optimizing global assets to respond to a pandemic viral outbreak, and this model could inform the pathway for influenza preparedness. The global network of influenza centers of excellence could advance progress on this pathway by increasing collaboration and expanding to ensure capacity building in LMICs. The sustainable financial vehicles discussed above would encourage and support LMICs in financing vaccine manufacturers to carry out R&D for seasonal and pandemic influenza vaccines.

Global Changes to Regulatory Systems to Improve Preparedness

During the COVID-19 pandemic, regulatory systems laid out clear requirements and worked together with industry partners in sharing data. In so doing, they facilitated overlapping preclinical and clinical phase studies, which resulted in the rapid development of novel vaccines directed at SARS-CoV-2 (Excler et al., 2021). However, pandemic influenza vaccines would ideally be developed even more rapidly, particularly for a potentially deadlier strain. To aid this process, clear guidelines need to be developed for preclinical and clinical studies to be performed in the interpandemic period.

Based on the results of clinical studies conducted for next-generation vaccines for seasonal influenza, then, regulators need to develop pathways for the rapid review of pandemic strain vaccines. These pathways could involve some interpandemic studies, such as phase I and II studies. Results of seasonal influenza studies suggest the possibility that a pandemic response may require only a strain change and demonstration of correlates of protection, followed by postauthorization confirmation of effectiveness.

Likewise, regulators need to develop clear pathways for the development of new vaccine platforms for seasonal influenza that are designed to generate data on multiple correlates of protection, efficacy, and safety. Given the crucial importance of data sharing between industry and regulators, regulators also need to develop protocols for these processes, as well as for chemistry, manufacturing, and control process inspections. Prepopulated regulatory assessment protocols with standardized endpoints and selection of sites at risk would support these efforts. Preparing such protocols before a pandemic occurs would allow for rapid development of high-quality vaccines. Early discussions with regulators and WHO are critical for the development of such protocols. During COVID-19, CEPI created an advisory group to communicate challenges from the regulators to work through regulatory challenges (CEPI, 2020). CEPI has also urged vaccine developers to use international standards for testing of efficacy, which is essential to establish correlates of protection. Additionally, CEPI engaged with academic journals to insist on the use of international standards for publishing. Together, these measures can streamline vaccine development with high standards.

Even though some effort was made to include more diverse populations in clinical trials for COVID-19 vaccines, diversity remained limited. For instance, pregnant individuals and children younger than 16 years were not included in initial clinical trials (Hwang et al., 2020; Subbaraman, 2021; Van Spall, 2021), while minority populations and the elderly were underrepresented (Flores et al., 2021). Therefore, regulators need to develop guidance for pandemic vaccine development for subpopulations at risk, including children, pregnant individuals, elderly people, and those with comorbidities.

Regulatory capacity also needs to be increased globally to support the rapid development of vaccines. WHO could act as a coordinator for the sharing of data among regulators, including data on efficacy and safety, postmarketing surveillance data, and product issues. With increased regulatory capacity and collaboration, core global regulatory standards of Emergency Use Authorization can support the development of a strong, stable global vaccine supply.

The COVID-19 pandemic showed the importance of clear and transparent public communications for vaccine acceptance in populations. Reduced trust and credibility among the public were the result of multiple factors, including a lack of transparency in the dissemination of data regarding the safety and risk of various vaccine candidates and results of risk–benefit analyses, along with the politicization of vaccine development. To address these issues, regulators and the industry could adopt a set of practices throughout the life cycle of vaccine development to ensure the transparency of data, including the release of trial data. It is essential for all communications to be based on science and as independent as possible of commercial and political interests. Improvement of diversity and inclusion in studies can aid in the communication to the population. In coordination with trusted scientific leaders, national regulators could advance clear and transparent public communications by collaborating on a global level to establish a coordinated communication capacity aimed at helping the public understand differences in recommendations in regions for the same vaccine across countries and regions. Community advisors could gather information and work together with regulators to provide guidance and real-time feedback on communication.

Global Coordination and Cooperation

CEPI and funding from the Wellcome Trust and the Bill & Melinda Gates Foundation were essential to the development of vaccines for COVID-19 using new platforms. CEPI was established to develop rapid-response platforms for new diseases with the potential to cause pandemics. The inclusion of MERS-CoV on its priority list helped prepare for the COVID-19 pandemic. CEPI began supporting vaccine development in January 2020 and had a diversified portfolio with established and novel technologies (CEPI, 2020). It additionally supported the R&D efforts by developing robust assays for determining a vaccine's immunogenicity. CEPI and other groups have also been tracking virus variants to determine their potential effect on vaccine effectiveness. The COVAX response facilitated unprecedented access to funds, but may benefit from measures to improve sustainability to account for future influenza outbreaks. CEPI's approach to addressing the COVID-19 pandemic provides a valuable model for how to effectively mobilize and optimize global assets to address a pandemic virus outbreak. This model could be used to address future pandemic influenza outbreaks (see Figure 6-1). However, one significant disadvantage of this model is that CEPI does not provide access to its assay protocols for early phase trials, and consequently limits reproducibility of assays. This disadvantage should be addressed in developing a sustainable model for addressing future outbreaks. An optimal harmonized framework for clinical development of vaccines for influenza would require coordinated funding for clinical trials that include diverse populations and are distributed globally. Manufacturing and fill and finish facilities would need to be expanded globally to allow early equitable access to vaccines. Global standards, based on regulatory standards, would support coordinated vaccine effectiveness and safety surveillance, providing a comprehensive and robust picture of these vital dimensions of all vaccines.

RECOMMENDATIONS

With the above priority needs in mind, the committee formulated recommendations in the dimensions of basic and translational science, clinical science, manufacturing science, and regulatory science (see Figure 6-2).

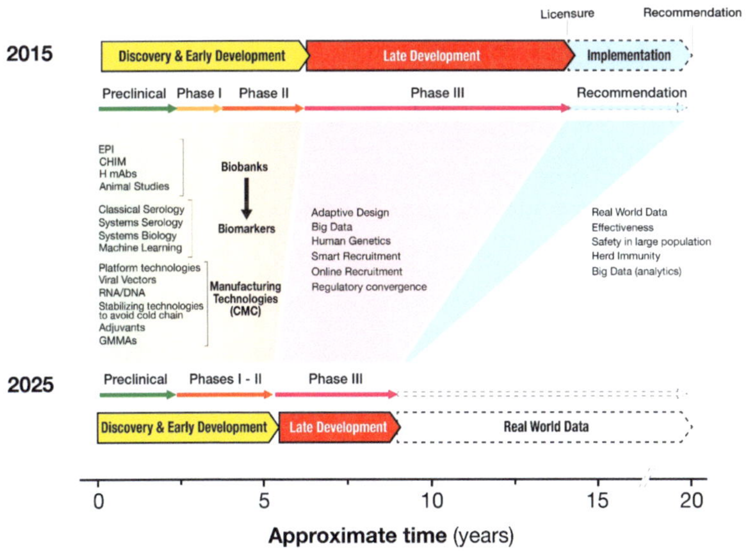

FIGURE 6-1 The future of pandemic vaccine development.
SOURCE: Black et al., 2020.

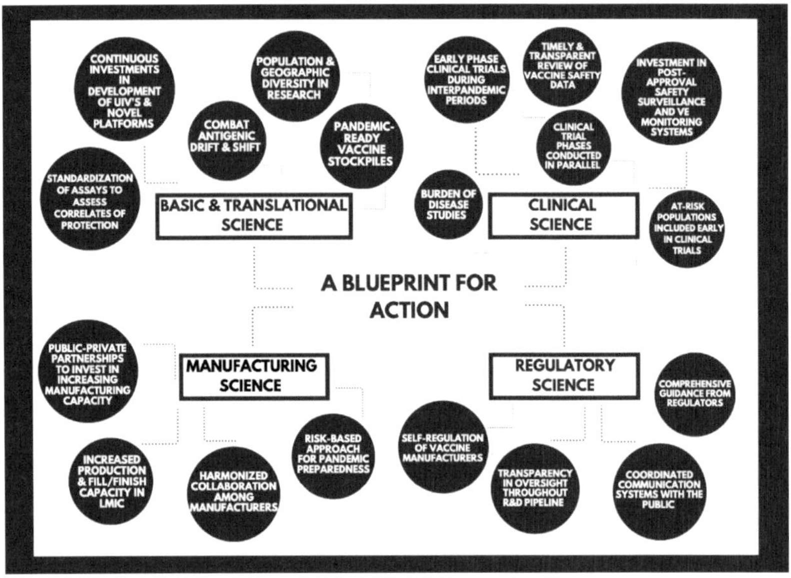

FIGURE 6-2 A blueprint for action.
NOTE: LMIC = low- and middle-income country; R&D = research and development; UIV = universal influenza vaccines.

Basic and Translational Science

Recommendation 2-1: The U.S. Department of Health and Human Services, through the National Institute of Allergy and Infectious Diseases, the Biomedical Advanced Research and Development Authority, and the U.S. Department of Defense, as well as other corresponding governmental and funding agencies domestically and abroad, should invest, proportionate to the enormous costs of pandemics, in basic and translational research to reveal a diverse array of influenza vaccines, using different platforms, viral targets, adjuvants, and delivery systems. This will allow selection of the candidates most fit for purpose to be brought to authorization and sufficient production and distribution to optimize the control of influenza across diverse settings and phases of pandemics and epidemics.

Recommendation 2-2: The World Health Organization should advocate and coordinate with multilateral stakeholders (e.g., the Coalition for Epidemic Preparedness Innovations), governments, funding agencies, the vaccine industry, and philanthropic organizations to build global capacity for robust and internationally comparable preclinical,

clinical, and immunological assessments of influenza vaccine candidates, including novel candidates that use innovative structures, targets, and delivery systems to potentially broaden or improve protection.

Recommendation 2-3: International research networks (e.g., the National Institutes of Health/U.S. Centers for Disease Control and Prevention funding networks) supported by governments and funding agencies, the World Health Organization, and the vaccine industry should support, carefully plan, and conduct multi-center international clinical trials and field studies to compare emerging vaccines with standard vaccines in, among others, geographically, demographically, and immunologically diverse populations to inform rational and situation-based use and manufacture of an extended array of vaccines.

Recommendation 2-4: National regulators should engage with the vaccine industry and academic researchers in the development, standardization, and implementation of innovative assays to evaluate vaccines that induce immunity through mechanisms other than strain-specific neutralizing hemagglutination-inhibiting antibodies in order to reach consensus on the validation of these assays that will allow approval or licensure of influenza vaccines based on a broader range of assays that reflect induction of immunity.

Clinical Science

Recommendation 3-1: The World Health Organization, in collaboration with national public health agencies (e.g., the U.S. Centers for Disease Control and Prevention, the European Centre for Disease Prevention and Control, the China Center for Disease Control and Prevention, and the Africa Centres for Disease Control and Prevention) should conduct burden-of-disease studies in low- and middle-income countries to understand factors such as the health and economic burden of influenza illness and barriers to immunization in adult, pregnant, and pediatric populations to ensure development of infrastructure and capacity needed for pandemic vaccine development and implementation. Cost–benefit analyses should include additional economic productivity losses caused by delayed access to a vaccine in a pandemic.

Recommendation 3-2: The International Coalition of Medicines Regulatory Authorities and the World Health Organization, in partnership with national regulatory (e.g., the U.S. Food and Drug Administration and the European Medicines Agency) and public health agencies (e.g., the U.S. Centers for Disease Control and Prevention, the European Centre for Disease Prevention and Control, the China Center for Disease Control and Prevention, and the Africa Centres for Disease Control and Prevention) should invest, on a global level, in data infrastructure and capacity building to conduct real-time sentinel site surveillance of vaccine safety and effectiveness of different vaccine products deployed for use in epidemics and pandemics in diverse populations (e.g., age group, gender, race/ethnicity, geographic, presence of comorbidities, pregnancy, and socioeconomics) including a plan to ensure coordination, collaboration, and data sharing across these sentinel surveillance sites.

Recommendation 3-3: The International Coalition of Medicines Regulatory Authorities and the World Health Organization (Global Advisory Committee on Vaccine Safety) should ensure international coordination and collaboration on the timely and transparent review of vaccine safety data during epidemics and pandemics to support real-time decision making about the use of vaccines. Safety data should be made available to support country-level benefit–risk assessments, particularly for low- and middle-income countries relying on regional data from sentinel sites conducting safety surveillance.

Manufacturing Science

Recommendation 4-1: The U.S. Department of Health and Human Services and the World Health Organization should develop a plan for a sufficient and self-sustainable global supply of influenza vaccines for pandemics. This includes

- Convening, supporting, and encouraging multi-national, public, and private vaccine manufacturers to benchmark, prioritize, and harmonize influenza vaccine manufacturing; and
- Enhancing and expanding support of the global influenza vaccine manufacturing network, creating manufacturing hubs for greater collaboration, and building capacity to address challenges in manufacturing in low- and middle-income countries.

Recommendation 4-2: Vaccine manufacturers should take a risk-based approach to pandemic influenza preparedness. This approach would be most effective if incentivized, and could include

- Participating during research and development, data sharing, technology adoption, and training activities with international partners;
- Expanding internal capacity to assess the production needs and their risks;

- Using scientific evidence to design strategies to reduce risks (e.g., World Health Organization prequalification, licensing, and marketing); and
- Formalizing technology transfer (scale-up and scale-out) activities taking into consideration timelines and the outcomes for equitable costs, access, and distribution.

Regulatory Science

Recommendation 5-1: The U.S. Food and Drug Administration and other national regulators (e.g., European Medicines Agency) working with the scientific community and pharmaceutical industry should enhance comprehensive guidance for the development of influenza vaccines on novel platforms through Emergency Use Authorization to full licensure. This guidance should provide pathways for seasonal and pandemic influenza.

Recommendation 5-2: The U.S. Food and Drug Administration and other national regulators (e.g., European Medicines Agency) should commit to transparency in the oversight of clinical trials, review of data, authorization, and approval of pandemic influenza vaccines, including the release of facility inspection findings, clinical trial protocols, and clinical data that are the basis of decision making. Regulators should convene independent advisory committees to systematically review data, make recommendations, and build public understanding and confidence prior to the authorization or approval of novel vaccines.

Recommendation 5-3: The World Health Organization and the International Coalition of Medicines Regulatory Authorities should encourage and support the coordination between regulatory and public health agencies (e.g., the U.S. Centers for Disease Control and Prevention, the European Centre for Disease Prevention and Control, the China Center for Disease Control and Prevention, and the Africa Centres for Disease Control and Prevention) when announcing different decisions on the same or similar vaccines, to explain the different underlying circumstances and judgments.

Recommendation 5-4: Vaccine manufacturers should adopt a code of conduct for press releases and other communications regarding vaccine trial results and other matters that emphasizes the critical role of regulatory review.

REFERENCES

Bender, E. 2019. Accelerating flu protection. *Nature* 573(7774):S60–S61.

Black, S., D. E. Bloom, D. C. Kaslow, S. Pecetta, and R. Rappuoli. 2020. Transforming vaccine development. *Seminars in Immunology* 50:101413.

CEPI (Coalition for Epidemic Preparedness Innovations). 2020. *2020 annual progress report: Covering the period from 1 January - 31 December.* Oslo, Norway: CEPI.

CIDRAP (Center for Infectious Disease Research and Policy). 2021. *Influenza vaccines roadmap*. https://www.cidrap.umn.edu/ongoing-programs/influenza-vaccines-roadmap (accessed October 19, 2021).

Excler, J.-L., M. Saville, S. Berkley, and J. H. Kim. 2021. Vaccine development for emerging infectious diseases. *Nature Medicine* 27(4):591–600.

Flores, L. E., W. R. Frontera, M. P. Andrasik, C. del Rio, A. Mondríguez-González, S. A. Price, E. M. Krantz, S. A. Pergam, and J. K. Silver. 2021. Assessment of the inclusion of racial/ethnic minority, female, and older individuals in vaccine clinical trials. *JAMA Network Open* 4(2):e2037640.

Gerdil, C. 2003. The annual production cycle for influenza vaccine. *Vaccine* 21(16):1776–1779.

Hwang, T. J., A. G. Randolph, and F. T. Bourgeois. 2020. Inclusion of children in clinical trials of treatments for coronavirus disease 2019 (COVID-19). *JAMA Pediatrics* 174(9):825–826.

Hyder, A. A., M. A. Hyder, K. Nasir, and P. Ndebele. 2021. Inequitable COVID-19 vaccine distribution and its effects. *Bulletin of the World Health Organization* 99(6):406.

Ortiz, J. R., and K. M. Neuzil. 2019. Influenza immunization in low- and middle-income countries: Preparing for next-generation influenza vaccines. *Journal of Infectious Diseases* 219(Suppl 1):S97–S106.

Rajaram, S., C. Boikos, D. K. Gelone, and A. Gandhi. 2020. Influenza vaccines: The potential benefits of cell-culture isolation and manufacturing. *Therapeutic Advances in Vaccines and Immunotherapy* 8:2515135520908121.

Sparrow, E., J. G. Wood, C. Chadwick, A. T. Newall, S. Torvaldsen, A. Moen, and G. Torelli. 2021. Global production capacity of seasonal and pandemic influenza vaccines in 2019. *Vaccine* 39(3):512–520.

Subbaraman, N. 2021. Pregnancy and COVID: What the data say. *Nature* 591(7849):193–195.

Van Spall, H. G. C. 2021. Exclusion of pregnant and lactating women from COVID-19 vaccine trials: A missed opportunity. *European Heart Journal* ehab103.

Williams, S. R., A. J. Driscoll, H. M. LeBuhn, W. H. Chen, K. M. Neuzil, and J. R. Ortiz. 2021. National routine adult immunisation programmes among World Health Organization member states: An assessment of health systems to deploy COVID-19 vaccines. *Eurosurveillance* 26(17):2001195.

Appendix A

Committee Biographies

Enriqueta Bond, Ph.D., M.A. (*Co-Chair*), served as the president of the Burroughs Wellcome Fund and was the executive officer of the Institute of Medicine. Currently she is a founding partner in QE Philanthropic Advisors that provides consulting services to nonprofits on organizational structure and function. Dr. Bond's degrees were in molecular biology and genetics; however, the bulk of her career has been addressing science and health policy and the role of philanthropy in support of biomedical research. She received her bachelor's degree from Wellesley College in 1961, her M.A. from the University of Virginia in 1963, and her Ph.D. in molecular biology and genetics from Georgetown University in 1969. Dr. Bond chaired the Board on African Science Academy and has served on a number of National Academies of Sciences, Engineering, and Medicine committees, most recently chairing studies on temporomandibular disorders and on reopening K–12 schools during the COVID-19 pandemic. She is a past member of the National Academies' Report Review Committee and has served on numerous government advisory groups including for the U.S. Centers for Disease Control and Prevention and the National Institutes of Health. She is a recipient of numerous honors including the 2008 Order of the Long Leaf Pine award, a fellow of the American Association for the Advancement of Science, and alumna of the year at Wellesley College.

Kanta Subbarao, M.B.B.S., M.P.H. (*Co-Chair*), was appointed the director of the World Health Organization (WHO) Collaborating Centre for Reference and Research on Influenza in 2016. Prior to her arrival in Melbourne, she was the chief of the Emerging Respiratory Viruses Section of the Laboratory of Infectious Diseases at the National Institute of Allergy and Infectious Diseases (NIAID) at the National Institutes of Health (NIH) in the United States from 2002 to 2016, and the chief of the Molecular Genetics Section of the Influenza Branch at the U.S. Centers for Disease Control and Prevention from 1997 to 2002. Ms. Kanta is a virologist and a physician with specialty training in pediatrics and pediatric infectious diseases. She received her M.B.B.S. from Christian Medical College, Vellore, in India; completed training in pediatrics and pediatric infectious diseases in the United States, and earned an M.P.H. in epidemiology from the University of Oklahoma Health Sciences Center. She received postdoctoral training in virology and vaccine development in the Laboratory of Infectious Diseases at NIAID. Over the years, her research has focused on newly emerging viral diseases of global importance including seasonal and pandemic influenza, severe acute respiratory syndrome, Middle East respiratory syndrome and now, SARS coronavirus 2 (SARS-CoV-2). Her current research efforts are directed at understanding the biology and immune responses to influenza viruses and vaccines and SARS-CoV-2. She is an internationally recognized leader in the field of emerging respiratory viruses. She is an elected fellow of the American Academy of Microbiology and the Infectious Diseases Society of America and is a member of the American Society of Microbiology, the American Society for Virology, and the Australasian Virology Society. In her current position as the director of the WHO Collaborating Centre for Reference and Research on Influenza, she advises WHO on viruses to be included in annual seasonal influenza vaccines.

Maria Elena Bottazzi, Ph.D., is the associate dean of the National School of Tropical Medicine, a professor of pediatrics and the co-director of the Texas Children's Center for Vaccine Development at the Baylor College of Medicine in Houston, Texas. She is an internationally recognized vaccine scientist and global health advocate with more than two decades of contributions in science, biotechnology, and vaccine development tackling neglected and emerging infectious diseases. As a global thought leader she has received national and international highly regarded awards, has more than 180 scientific papers, and participated in more than 250 conferences worldwide. In 2020, *Forbes* selected her as one of 100 Most Powerful Women in Central America. Dr. Bottazzi is a member of the National Academy of Science of Honduras and an Emerging Leader in Health and Medicine Scholar of the National Academy of Medicine in the United States. Currently she serves as the co-chair of the Vaccines and Therapeutics Taskforce of the Lancet Commission on COVID-19. Dr. Bottazzi obtained her bachelor's degree in microbiology and clinical chemistry from the National Autonomous University of Honduras and a doctorate in molecular immunology and experimental pathology from the University of Florida.

Her postdoctoral training in cellular biology was completed at the University of Miami and the University of Pennsylvania.

Rebecca J. Cox, Ph.D., is a professor of medical virology and the head of the Influenza Centre at the University of Bergen and Haukeland University Hospital, Norway, leading a team of 15 scientists. She has more than 25 years of experience of influenza work particularly in development and evaluation of influenza vaccines. She has serves as an advisor to the World Health Organization SAGE Immunization Working Group on Influenza and the European Medicines Agency. She is the deputy chair of influenza and other respiratory viruses and the senior editor for the journal *Influenza and Other Respiratory Viruses* and the associate editor of the journals *Human Vaccines* and *Immunotherapeutics and Vaccines*. Her research focuses on epidemics and pandemics with particular focus on human immune responses after infection and vaccination.

Annette Fox, Ph.D., is an immunologist with specialist expertise and knowledge in research on influenza, including laboratory, epidemiological, and clinical studies. She is a senior research scientist with the World Health Organization's Collaborating Centre for Reference and Research on Influenza and holds honorary senior fellow appointments at the University of Melbourne (Australia). Dr. Fox studied fundamental aspects of gamma delta T cells (receptor use and biology) for her Ph.D. at the University of Melbourne. This was followed by a postdoc at the Walter and Eliza Hall Institute (Melbourne, Australia) where she initiated novel research on innate immune recognition of transplants, and 3 years with the Medical Research Council in the Gambia investigating immunity against tuberculosis. In 2008, she joined the Oxford University Clinical Research Unit in Vietnam, and undertook pioneering research on influenza and dengue immunity, pathogenesis, and transmission. Dr. Fox returned to Australia in 2014, and has established a research platform to understand how serological responses to influenza are influenced by prior exposures and may be enhanced to improve vaccine outcomes. Her research platform revolves around longitudinal community and hospital-based cohorts that investigate influenza vaccinations and infections. Her lab has developed a series of tools to dissect antibody and B cell responses to influenza in these cohorts, and to model interactions with exposure history. High throughput serology and computational analysis are combined with virus reverse engineering to quantify the influenza strain coverage of antibodies induced. B cells are analyzed using influenza-protein probes in 20+ color flow cytometry, as well as B cell receptor sequencing and recombinant mAb generation. Her work has helped to establish the need for extended serological analysis of influenza vaccine responses, and for greater understanding of how prior influenza exposures affect vaccine responses.

Florian Krammer, Ph.D., is a professor of vaccinology in the Department of Microbiology at the Icahn School of Medicine at Mount Sinai. Dr. Krammer has published more than 250 papers and is a peer reviewer for more than 30 journals. He has focused on the development of broadly neutralizing anti-hemagglutinin stalk antibodies and the design of a universal influenza virus vaccine. The Krammer laboratory, which is also part of the National Institutes of Health–funded Centers for Excellence in Influenza Research and Surveillance, focuses on understanding broadly reactive immune responses against the surface glycoproteins of RNA viruses such as influenza with the goal to develop better vaccines and novel therapeutics. Professor Krammer received his advanced training in biotechnology and applied virology at the University of Natural Resources and Life Sciences, Vienna (Mentor: Dr. Reingard Grabherr), where he gained extensive experience with expression and purification of recombinant (glyco-) proteins and influenza virus-like particles. He established various expression systems for these proteins using insect cells/baculovirus, mammalian cells, bacteria, yeast, and plants. Furthermore, he worked on a novel influenza virus rescue system based on baculovirus transduction of mammalian cells and a novel bioassay to measure inhibition of the influenza virus polymerase complex by cap-snatching inhibitors. He graduated from the University of Natural Resources and Life Sciences, Vienna, in 2010.

Grace M. Lee, M.D., M.P.H., is a professor of pediatrics at the Stanford University School of Medicine. She has earned distinction through her research and policy leadership to avert harm from infectious diseases. Her body of work has had national impact on public health policy for vaccines and hospital-acquired infections. Her talent and skills in large-scale informatics were key to the development of near real-time safety surveillance for H1N1 vaccine via the nation's largest active vaccine monitoring networks sponsored by the U.S. Centers for Disease Control and Prevention (U.S. CDC) and the U.S. Food and Drug Administration. Dr. Lee's seminal research in hospital-acquired infections has generated a number of high-impact findings. Dr. Lee's accomplishments and ability to integrate the ideas of experts from multiple disciplines have led to invitations to multiple leadership roles. These include election to the boards of the Society for Healthcare Epidemiology of America and the Pediatric Infectious Diseases Society; a member of the National Academies of Sciences, Engineering, and Medicine's Board on Population Health and Public Health Practice (2013–2019); and the current chair of U.S. CDC's Advisory Committee on Immunization Practices, the nation's leading policy-making group for vaccines. She is currently a member of the ACIP COVID-19 vaccines workgroup, the chair of the COVID-19 Vaccine Safety Technical (VaST) workgroup, and a member of the Western States Scientific Safety Review Committee. VaST reviews safety data from all federal safety surveillance systems on a weekly basis for COVID-19 vaccines and supports the ACIP decision making regarding the continued use of COVID-19 vaccines for the United States.

John C. Martin, Ph.D., M.B.A., was the former executive chair and the chief executive officer of Gilead Sciences. Dr. Martin previously served as Gilead's vice president for research and development and chair. He previously worked at Syntax Corporation and was the director of antiviral chemistry at Bristol Myers Squibb. While working at Gilead Sciences his focus was on anti-HIV medications and AIDS prevention through pre-exposure prophylaxis. He developed the first single tablet treatment for HIV and expanded access to HIV and hepatitis C treatments in developing countries, earning him the Lifetime Achievement Award for Public Service and the Biotechnology Heritage Award.

Joshua M. Sharfstein, M.D., is the vice dean for public health practice and community engagement and a professor of the practice in health policy and management at the Johns Hopkins Bloomberg School of Public Health. He is also the director of the Bloomberg American Health Initiative. Previously, Dr. Sharfstein served as the secretary of the Maryland Department of Health and Mental Hygiene, as the principal deputy commissioner of the U.S. Food and Drug Administration, and as the health commissioner of Baltimore City. In these positions, he pursued creative solutions to long-standing challenges, including drug overdose deaths, infant mortality, unsafe consumer products, and school failure. He is an elected member of the National Academy of Medicine and a fellow of the National Academy of Public Administration.

Milagritos D. Tapia, M.D. Dr. Tapia's research focuses primarily on the epidemiology of vaccine-preventable diseases in Mali and the development of vaccines to address these diseases. In conjunction with the team at CVD-Mali (Centre pour le Developpement des Vaccins–Mali), she has conducted and participated in the following vaccine development activities: (1) a pivotal vaccine trial that demonstrated the efficacy of live, oral, pentavalent rotavirus vaccine (Rotateq) in Africa; (2) a large trial of trivalent influenza vaccine, administered to pregnant Malian women, demonstrated its efficacy in the prevention of influenza in the infants up to 6 months of age; and (3) a first trial in humans of a candidate vaccine against Ebolavirus and phase II trials of a candidate vaccine against Ebolavirus in Malian adults and children. Dr. Tapia is the principal investigator in clinical research relating to meningococcal vaccine that is supported by Walvax Technology Ltd.

Appendix B

Disclosure of Unavoidable Conflict of Interest

The conflict of interest policy of the National Academies of Sciences, Engineering, and Medicine (http://www.nationalacademies.org/coi) prohibits the appointment of an individual to a committee authoring a Consensus Study Report if the individual has a conflict of interest that is relevant to the task to be performed. An exception to this prohibition is permitted if the National Academies determines that the conflict is unavoidable and the conflict is publicly disclosed. A determination of a conflict of interest for an individual is not an assessment of that individual's actual behavior or character or ability to act objectively despite the conflicting interest.

Dr. Florian Krammer has a conflict of interest in relation to his service on the Committee on Vaccine Research and Development Recommendations for Advancing Pandemic and Seasonal Influenza Vaccine Preparedness and Response because he has consulting relationships with the vaccine manufacturing companies Avimex and Seqirus.

The National Academies has concluded that in order for the committee to accomplish the tasks for which it was established, its membership must include at least one person with current experience in biotechnology, novel vaccine platforms, and applied industry experience in vaccine research and development. As described in his biographical summary, Dr. Krammer has extensive current experience in leveraging novel technologies to develop vaccines and direct experience working with influenza manufacturing companies developing practical and effective vaccine platforms.

Appendix C

Staff and Consultant Biographies

STAFF

Hoda Soltani, Ph.D., M.P.H., is this study's director and a program officer with the Board on Global Health. She received her Ph.D. in nutritional biology from the University of California, Davis. She completed her research at the Western Human Nutrition Research Center, a division of the U.S. Department of Agriculture, where she examined the interrelationships of nutrition, physiological stress, and cardiometabolic outcomes in overweight women. She also received her M.P.H. from the University of Toronto in 2011 and her B.Sc. in human ecology from the University of Western Ontario in 2009. Professionally, she has more than a decade of experience working as a scientist and a project manager in a myriad of diverse settings, including academia, industry, clinical care, and public health organizations.

Emilie Ryan-Castillo is a senior program assistant with the Board on Global Health, working on the influenza consensus studies. She has a B.S. in public health from American University. In the past, she was a program assistant at FHI 360 and worked on diabetes prevention and childhood obesity research projects. In this role, she helped execute several large meetings bringing together the top researchers from the U.S. Centers for Disease Control and Prevention, the National Institutes of Health, the U.S. Department of Agriculture, and the Robert Wood Johnson Foundation for the National Collaborative on Childhood Obesity Research. Recently, she served as a Rural Community Health Volunteer in the Peace Corps Benin, where she worked on improving maternal health, vaccination rates, and community outreach at a local clinic in the Borgou Department.

Elizabeth Ashby, M.S., is a research associate with the Board on Global Health. She holds a master's degree in environmental science from George Mason University, with a focus on risk factors for zoonotic disease transmission. Previously, she has conducted research in collaboration with the PREDICT project for global disease surveillance to assess risk factors for zoonotic disease transmission in Kenya. She has also worked with a private consulting company to apply social marketing interventions and innovative technologies to pressing global health issues. Her primary interests include applying a One Health lens to analyze challenges related to emerging pandemic threats.

Hannah K. Collins is an independent consultant for SGNL Solutions and supports the work of the National Academies as a research associate, advising on and editing reports, authoring committee meeting proceedings, and conducting supplemental research. She also works as a science writer for SGNL Solutions, authoring and editing academic workshop proceedings. She graduated from St. Lawrence University with a B.S in neuroscience and is working toward her M.S. in neuroscience at the City University of London where she is interested in public health and neurodegenerative disease research.

Patricia A. Cuff, M.S., M.P.H., is a senior program officer with the Board on Global Health where she directs the Global Forum on Innovation in Health Professional Education—a position she has held since 2012. Ms. Cuff is also leading the U.S. Food and Drug Administration–funded study looking at mutual recognition agreements in the regulation of medicines, and a special COVID-related project with select academies in Africa. Ms. Cuff worked for 11 years on the African Science Academy Development Initiative where she was the country liaison to the Uganda National Academy of Sciences. She has directed and co-directed multiple studies at the National Academies including clinical trials during the 2014–2015 Ebola outbreak, options for overseas placement of U.S. health professionals, and enhancing the behavioral and social science content of medical school curricula. Ms. Cuff joined the National Academies staff to work on the report *Emerging Microbial Threats to Health in the 21st Century*. Before coming to Washington, DC, she worked at St. Luke's—Roosevelt Hospital Center in New York City in the field of HIV nutrition as a counselor, researcher, and lecturer on topics of adult and pediatric HIV. She received her M.S. in nutrition and her M.P.H. in population and family health from Columbia University, and performed her undergraduate studies at the University of Connecticut.

Julie A. Pavlin, M.D., Ph.D., M.P.H., is the senior director of the Board on Global Health and is board certified in preventive medicine and public health. She is a retired Colonel in the U.S. Army with previous assignments including the Armed Forces Research Institute of Medical Sciences in Bangkok, Thailand; the Walter Reed Army Institute of Research; and the U.S. Army Medical Research Institute for Infectious Diseases. After she retired from active duty, she served as the deputy director, Armed Forces Health Surveillance Center. She concentrated most of her time with the U.S. Department of Defense in the design of real-time disease surveillance systems and was a co-founder of the International Society for Disease Surveillance.

CONSULTANT

Maartje Wouters, Ph.D., M.S., is a freelance medical and a science writer. She obtained an M.Sc. in human pathobiology and toxicology from the Radboud University in Nijmegen, the Netherlands, and a Ph.D. in cancer immunology from the University of Groningen, the Netherlands. Subsequently, she completed postdoctoral training in cancer immunotherapy at BC Cancer in Victoria, BC. The focus of her research was therapeutic targets in the immune environment of ovarian cancer. With more than 8 years of experience in preclinical research in immunology and oncology, Dr. Wouters now works as a medical and science writer developing protocols, reports, and other documentation for academia, industry, government, and nongovernmental organizations.

Appendix D

Public Meeting Agendas

Committee on Vaccine Research and Development for Advancing Pandemic and Seasonal Influenza Preparedness and Response

First Committee Meeting Agenda

March 8 and 10, 2021
Orientation and Conflict of Interest Discussion: March 8, 7:00–9:30 PM EST
Speaker Session: March 10, 7:00–10:00 AM EST
Planning/Working Session: March 10, 3:30–6:30 PM EST
Virtual

Meeting Objectives

- Conduct committee and staff introductions
- Orient the committee to the National Academies consensus study process
- Conduct the bias and conflict of interest discussion
- Hold on open session to hear from sponsoring agency on its perspective of the Statement of Task and to hear from relevant stakeholders
- Discuss the Statement of Task and work plan and agree on approach to completing the task
- Identify information needs and future meeting topics

Monday, March 8, 2021

7:30–8:30 PM EST CLOSED SESSION—COMMITTEE MEMBERS ONLY

8:30–9:00 PM EST OPEN SESSION

8:30 PM **Sponsor Perspective on Charge to the Committee**

8:45 PM **Q&A for Sponsor**

9:00–9:30 PM EST CLOSED SESSION—COMMITTEE MEMBERS ONLY

9:30 PM **Adjourn**

Wednesday, March 10, 2021

7:00–9:00 AM EST OPEN SESSION

7:00 AM **Welcome and Opening Remarks**

7:10 AM **COVID-19 Response: Lessons Learned**
NADINE ROUPHAEL
Department of Medicine, Division of Infectious Diseases
Emory University School of Medicine

7:30 AM **Discussion with Committee**

7:45 AM **Regulatory Pathways in the United States to Facilitate Vaccine Availability**
PETER MARKS
Center for Biologics Evaluation and Research
U.S. Food and Drug Administration

8:00 AM **Discussion with Committee**

8:10 AM **Break**

8:15 AM	**Overview of the Influenza Vaccines R&D Roadmap and the Universal Influenza Vaccine Technology Landscape** JULIE OSTROWSKY Center for Infectious Disease Research and Policy University of Minnesota
8:40 AM	**Discussion with Committee**
8:55 AM	**Break**

9:00–10:00 AM EST CLOSED SESSION—COMMITTEE MEMBERS ONLY

10:00 AM	**Adjourn Morning Session**

Wednesday, March 10, 2021

3:30–6:30 PM EST CLOSED SESSION

Second Committee Meeting

March 30, 2021
3:00–6:00 PM EST
Virtual

Meeting Objectives

- Review key discussion points of previous meeting
- Address the current state of basic/translational science of influenza vaccines
- Address the implications of "lessons learned" from COVID-19 on basic/translational science of influenza vaccines
- Discuss the potential application of emerging technologies to seasonal or pandemic influenza outbreaks
- Identify information needs and future meeting topics

March 30, 2021

3:00–4:30 PM EST OPEN SESSION

3:00 PM	**Welcome, Review of Previous Session**

3:10 PM	**Broadly Protective and Universal Influenza Virus Vaccines in Development** FLORIAN KRAMMER Professor in Vaccinology Department of Microbiology Icahn School of Medicine at Mount Sinai
3:25 PM	**Discussion with Committee**
3:35 PM	**Perspective on Lessons from the COVID-19 Vaccine Experience** BARNEY GRAHAM Deputy Director, Vaccine Research Center Chief, Viral Pathogenesis Laboratory and Translational Science Core National Institutes of Health
3:50 PM	**Discussion with Committee**
4:00 PM	**Vaccinating Against Influenza Viruses: Can New Memory Be Induced When Old Memory Is Recalled** ANNETTE FOX Senior Research Scientist World Health Organization Collaborating Centre for Reference and Research on Influenza University of Melbourne
4:15 PM	**Discussion with Committee**
4:25 PM	**Break, End of Open Session**

4:30–6:00 PM EST CLOSED SESSION—COMMITTEE MEMBERS ONLY

Third Committee Meeting

April 15, 2021
3:00–6:00 PM EST
Virtual

Meeting Objectives

- Review key discussion points of previous meeting
- Continue discussion of basic/translational science of vaccine research and development
- Identify priority goals for future research and development, including potential timelines and actors
- Discuss needs and mechanisms for global collaboration, highlighting issues of equity
- Identify information needs and future meeting topics

April 15, 2021

3:00–4:15 PM EST OPEN SESSION

3:00 PM **Welcome, Review of Previous Session**

3:10 PM **Overview of Novel Platforms in Influenza Vaccine and Integrating Lessons from COVID-19**
REBECCA COX
Professor of Medical Virology and Head of the Influenza Centre
University of Bergen

3:25 PM **Discussion with Committee**

3:35 PM **Lessons Learned from COVID-19 Vaccine Development**
MELANIE SEVILLE
Director of Vaccine Development
Coalition for Epidemic Preparedness Innovations

3:50 PM **Discussion with Committee**

4:10 PM **Break, End of Open Session**

4:15–6:00 PM EST CLOSED SESSION—COMMITTEE MEMBERS ONLY

Fourth Committee Meeting

April 28, 2021
3:00–6:00 PM EST
Virtual

Meeting Objectives

- Review key discussion points of previous meeting
- Address the current state of clinical science of influenza vaccines
- Address the implications of "lessons learned" from COVID-19 on clinical science of influenza vaccines
- Discuss the potential application of emerging technologies to seasonal or pandemic influenza outbreaks

April 28, 2021

3:00–3:20 PM EST CLOSED SESSION

3:20–4:30 PM EST OPEN SESSION

3:20 PM	**Introduction to Open Session**
3:30 PM	**Overview of Vaccine Clinical Trials in Lower- and Middle-Income Countries** MILAGRITOS TAPIA Professor of Pediatrics and Medicine University of Maryland at Baltimore
3:45 PM	**Discussion with Committee**
4:00 PM	**Influenza Vaccines in LMICs: Manufacturing and Feasibility Considerations** KATHY NEUZIL Director, Center for Vaccine Development University of Maryland School of Medicine

4:15 PM **Discussion with Committee**

4:25 PM **Break, End of Open Session**

4:30–6:00 PM EST CLOSED SESSION—COMMITTEE MEMBERS ONLY

Fifth Committee Meeting

May 12, 2021
8:00–11:00 AM EST
Virtual

Meeting Objectives

- Review key discussion points of previous meeting
- Continue discussion of clinical science of vaccine research and development
- Identify priority goals for future research and development, including potential timelines and actors
- Discuss needs and mechanisms for global collaboration, highlighting issues of equity
- Identify information needs and future meeting topics

May 12, 2021

8:00–9:30 AM EST OPEN SESSION

8:00 AM **Introduction to Open Session**

8:10 AM **Lessons from COVID-19 for Influenza Preparedness**
JEROME KIM
Director General
International Vaccine Institute

8:25 AM **Discussion with Committee**

8:35 AM	**Understanding Vaccine Effectiveness: Lessons from COVID-19 and Applications for Influenza** Ben Cowling Professor of Epidemiology and Biostatistics School of Public Health The University of Hong Kong
8:50 AM	**Discussion with Committee**
9:00 AM	**Successes and Challenges in Monitoring Vaccine Safety in the United States** Grace Lee Professor of Pediatrics Stanford University School of Medicine
9:30 AM	**Break, End of Open Session**

9:30–11:00 AM EST CLOSED SESSION—COMMITTEE MEMBERS ONLY

Sixth Committee Meeting

May 26, 2021
3:00–6:00 PM EST
Virtual

Meeting Objectives

- Address the current state of manufacturing and regulatory science of influenza vaccines
- Address the implications of "lessons learned" from COVID-19 on manufacturing and regulatory science of influenza vaccines
- Discuss the potential application of emerging technologies to seasonal and pandemic influenza outbreaks nationally and globally
- Identify conclusions and recommendations for best practices in manufacturing and regulatory science
- Identify information needs and future meeting topics

May 26, 2021

3:00–4:30 PM EST OPEN SESSION

3:00 PM	**Welcome, Review of Previous Session**
3:05 PM	**Successes in Technology Transfer and Manufacturing Partnerships: Lessons from COVID-19 and Applications for Influenza** MARIA ELENA BOTTAZI Associate Dean and Professor Baylor College of Medicine
3:15 PM	**Discussion with Committee**
3:25 PM	**Manufacturing Science of Influenza Vaccine Research and Development** ROBERT JOHNSON Director, Influenza and Emerging Infectious Diseases Division and COVID-19 Incident Manager Biomedical Advanced Research Development Authority
3:35 PM	**Discussion with Committee**
3:45 PM	**Developing Vaccines in the Era of Genomics** RINO RAPPUOLI Chief Scientist and Head of External Research and Development GlaxoSmithKline
3:55 PM	**Discussion with Committee**
4:05 PM	**Manufacturing Science of Influenza Vaccine R&D: Mind the Adjacencies** DAVID KASLOW Chief Scientific Officer PATH
4:15 PM	**Discussion with Committee**
4:30 PM	**Break, End of Open Session**

4:30 PM–6:00 PM EST CLOSED SESSION—COMMITTEE MEMBERS ONLY

Seventh Committee Meeting

June 10, 2021
3:00–6:00 PM EST
Virtual

Meeting Objectives

- Address the current state of regulatory science of influenza vaccines
- Address the implications of "lessons learned" from COVID-19 on regulatory science of influenza vaccines
- Discuss the potential application of emerging technologies to seasonal or pandemic influenza outbreaks nationally and globally
- Identify conclusions and recommendations for best practices in regulatory science

June 10, 2021

3:00–4:30 PM EST OPEN SESSION

3:00 PM	**Welcome**
3:10 PM	**Opening Remarks by Joshua Sharfstein**
3:15 PM	**Key Considerations for Vaccine Research and Development** Phil Dormitzer Vice President and Chief Scientific Officer: Viral Vaccines Pfizer Inc.
3:30 PM	**Key Considerations for Vaccine Research and Development** Rita Helfand Chair World Health Organization Global Advisory Committee for Vaccine Safety

3:25 PM	**Key Considerations for Vaccine Research and Development** NICOLE LURIE Director, Strategic Advisor to the Chief Executive Officer Coalition for Epidemic Preparedness Initiatives
3:30 PM	**Panel: Regulatory Science of Vaccine Development**
4:30 PM	**Break, End of Open Session**

4:30–6:00 PM EST CLOSED SESSION—COMMITTEE MEMBERS ONLY